Lacanian Psychoanalytic Writings

Lacanian Psychoanalytic Writings: The Littoral Word presents cutting-edge Lacanian psychoanalytic thought by leaders in the field.

Each chapter is written by authors who, in one way or another, take up Jacques Lacan's observation that each psychoanalysis invents psychoanalysis anew. They bring to the field not an orthodoxy but a rigorous singularity which continues to be pertinent to what Freud described as the malaise of civilisation. Megan Williams brings together important work by Jean Allouch, Christian Fierens and members of the Freudian School of Melbourne, exploring themes of madness, hysteria, sexuality and language through a Lacanian lens.

This essential collection will appeal to psychoanalysts, psychotherapists and psychiatrists. It will also be of interest to academics and scholars of philosophy, cultural studies, literature and linguistics who engage with psychoanalytic theory.

Megan Williams is a psychoanalyst of more than 30 years' standing, based in Australia. She is an Analyst of the School of the Freudian School of Melbourne and practises psychoanalysis in Melbourne as well as giving seminars. She has published numerous articles in psychoanalysis and has a particular interest in writing.

Papers of the Freudian School of Melbourne
Series Editor: Megan Williams

Other titles in the series:

Invention in the Real
Papers of the Freudian School of Melbourne, Volume 24
Edited by Linda Clifton

Since Lacan
Papers of the Freudian School of Melbourne, Volume 25
Edited by Linda Clifton

Lacan and Other Heresies: Lacanian Psychoanalytic Writings
Papers of the Freudian School of Melbourne, Volume 26
Edited by Linda Clifton

Lacanian Psychoanalytic Writings: The Littoral Word
Papers of the Freudian School of Melbourne, Volume 27
Edited by Megan Williams

For more information about this series, please visit: www.routledge.com/

Lacanian Psychoanalytic Writings

The Littoral Word

Edited by Megan Williams

Routledge
Taylor & Francis Group
LONDON AND NEW YORK

Designed cover image: Portrait de Jacques Lacan, psychiatre et psychanalyste en octobre 1967, en France. (Photo by Giancarlo BOTTI/Gamma-Rapho via Getty Images)

First published 2026
by Routledge
4 Park Square, Milton Park, Abingdon, Oxon OX14 4RN

and by Routledge
605 Third Avenue, New York, NY 10158

Routledge is an imprint of the Taylor & Francis Group, an informa business

British Library Cataloguing-in-Publication Data
A catalogue record for this book is available from the British Library

ISBN: 978-1-041-19607-5 (hbk)
ISBN: 978-1-041-19606-8 (pbk)
ISBN: 978-1-003-71248-0 (ebk)

DOI: 10.4324/9781003712480

Typeset in Times New Roman
by Apex CoVantage, LLC

Contents

About the editor and contributors

Jean Allouch was a psychoanalyst practising in Paris, a member of the École Freudienne de Paris until its dissolution in 1981, then a founding member of the École lacanienne de psychanalyse from 1985 until his death in 2023. He held a regular seminar at Saint Anne Hospital, Paris, and in Latin America. He published extensively in French, Spanish, Portuguese, German and English, and several of his papers appear in the *Papers of the Freudian School of Melbourne*. A series of lectures he presented at the University of Melbourne in 2004 were published in *Lacan Love Melbourne Seminars and Other Works* (Bookbound Publishers, 2007). He also created the collection *Les grand classiques de l'erotologie moderne* at Epel Éditions in an endeavour to take up feminist and queer theory and gay and lesbian studies as new fields that problematise the erotic in psychoanalysis (www.JeanAllouch.com).

Linda Clifton is an analyst and co-director of the Freudian School of Melbourne and the immediate past editor of the *Papers of the Freudian School of Melbourne*. She works as a psychoanalyst in private practice.

Christian Fierens is a psychoanalyst and psychiatrist based in Tervuren, Belgium. He obtained a PhD on the topic of psychosis in Freud's work and has published several books in which he interrogates the work of Freud and Lacan, including *The Soul of Narcissism*, *The Jouissance Principle*, and *A Reading of Anxiety: Lacan's Seminar X*, published by Routledge and translated into English.

Shubha Gokhale is a member of the Freudian School of Melbourne. Shubha works with children and adults in psychoanalytic private practice in Geelong and in a community-based organisation in Melbourne for refugees and asylum seekers. She has previously worked in schools and community health settings in India and Australia.

Peter Gunn is a psychoanalyst in private practice in Melbourne. He has published numerous psychoanalytic papers in *Papers of The Freudian School of Melbourne* and elsewhere.

Rodney Kleiman was a psychoanalyst who, until his death in 2024, was a co-director of the Freudian School of Melbourne and Analyst of the School. Originally trained as a psychiatrist, he worked predominantly in private practice with an ongoing appointment as a consultant with mental health services. He published numerous articles in the *Papers of the Freudian School of Melbourne* and presented at psychoanalytic seminars and conferences over many years. He had a particular interest in the questions posed by psychosis and its potential treatment.

Tine Nørregaard is a psychoanalyst in private practice in Melbourne and an Analyst Member of the Freudian School of Melbourne. She co-convenes the seminar 'In Consideration of Anguish' with Megan Williams. She has written numerous articles on theoretical and clinical psychoanalysis in English and in Danish and has translated articles from French to English. Some are published in the *Papers of the Freudian School of Melbourne* and *Écritique*, of which she was co-editor from 2000–2003. From 2007 to 2016 she co-convened the seminar 'Psychoanalysis and the Child' with Michael Gerard Plastow. She was previously associate lecturer at the Institute of Clinical Psychology and the Department of Philosophy, Education and Rhetoric, University of Copenhagen.

David Pereira is a psychoanalyst in private practice in Melbourne, Australia, where he is an Analyst of the School and is currently a co-director of the Freudian School of Melbourne. He has written numerous articles on theoretical and clinical psychoanalysis published in both the *Papers of the Freudian School of Melbourne* and elsewhere. He was formally consultant psychoanalyst with the Alfred Hospital Child and Adolescent Mental Health Service and senior clinician with the Department of Child Psychotherapy, Royal Children's Hospital, Melbourne.

Debbie Plastow is an Analyst Member of the Freudian School of Melbourne (School of Lacanian Psychoanalysis). She works at Austin Health's Booboop Narrkwarren Nagarra-jarra-noun (Statewide Child and Family Healing Centre) as a senior mental health clinician and in private practice.

Michael Gerard Plastow is an Analyst of the School of the Freudian School of Melbourne, practising in Melbourne. He is the author of *What Is a Child?: Childhood, Psychoanalysis, and Discourse*, published by Karnac in 2015, and *Sabina Spielrein: The Poetry of Psychoanalysis*, published by Routledge in 2019. Amongst his current projects is the co-editing and translating with Christiane Weller of a collection of all Sabina Spielrein's published psychoanalytical papers for the first time in English.

Sabina Spielrein (1885–1942) was an early psychoanalyst of Russian origin who had an analysis with Carl Gustav Jung in Zürich and later moved closer to Freud in her theoretical approach. She wrote mostly in German, and her works are notable for their detailed clinical observation of cases. She was an innovative thinker and psychoanalyst, in particular in her work with children, which began long before that of Melanie Klein and Anna Freud. She worked in Switzerland, Austria and Germany before returning to Russia in 1923. She was killed with her two daughters and thousands of other Jews in Rostov-on-Don by the occupying Nazi forces.

Christiane Weller is associate professor in European languages (German) at Monash University, Melbourne. She has published in the field of the medical humanities on psychoanalytic theory and psychiatric art collections and on psychosis and writing. She is a member of the Freudian School of Melbourne.

Megan Williams is an Analyst of the School of the Freudian School of Melbourne and practises psychoanalysis in Melbourne and Geelong. She is the current editor of the *Papers of the Freudian School of Melbourne* and co-convenor with Tine Nørregaard of the seminar 'In Consideration of Anguish.' She has presented and published numerous seminars and papers in PFSM and elsewhere.

Logos

Everything that is written stems from the fact that it will forever be impossible to write, as such, the sexual relationship. It is on that basis that there is a certain effect of discourse, which is called writing.[1]

We write in order to disturb language, to dislodge it from its familiar place.

To write in order to situate oneself differently in relation to the history that inhabits one. To speak in order to cultivate the strangeness of one's own language.

The psychotic speaks the truth—we are infected by the alien virus of language.

I have only one language. It is not mine.[2]

In the abstinence of the psychoanalytic clinic, it is only the word that can penetrate.

Through fleshing out the word . . . hysteria becomes psychoanalysis.

Aside from the first, which comes from Lacan's *Seminar XVII*, the writings above are all taken from the papers contained in this edition of the *Papers of the Freudian School of Melbourne*. Some are direct quotations; some are paraphrasings by me or even, therefore, parapraxes. In their variety, their varité, they examine the ways in which language is lived.

Some engage with writing—the manner in which the inexistence of that which we seek is transformed into a writing that disturbs language where it nestles in family and in history and makes it strange, arousing a kind of knowing that owes nothing to recognition.

Others come to grips with the fleshiness of speech, of words which have the potential to be realised in that strange sonority of the voice evoked in Shubha

1 Lacan, J. (2007 [1969–1970]). *The Other Side of Psychoanalysis: The Seminar of Jacques Lacan Book XVII*. J.-A. Miller (Ed.), R. Grigg (Trans.). New York & London: W. W. Norton & Co., pp. 34–35.

2 Derrida, J. (1998 [1996]). *Monolingualism of the Other; or, the Prosthesis of Origin*. P. Mensah (Trans.). Stanford: Stanford University Press, p. 1, cited in the chapter by Shubha Gokhale in this volume.

Gokhale's chapter, where a mother's tongue both tears the child away and also invades or makes holes in its flesh, necessitating a speaking which will thereafter hold foreignness within itself. Rodney Kleiman evokes the virus of language inhabiting us, testified to by the madman. David Pereira writes of words having the power to dis-organise a body into flesh that overflows the constraints of desire. Linda Clifton writes of words which penetrate, arousing jouissance in its most intimate relation with anguish. In Debbie Plastow's chapter, jouissance smooches with language in the symptom. Each chapter engages in some way with the manner in which language both constrains and gives passage to that real which hides, dissembles, commands, rants, believes, hates, loves or overflows in the ways which the authors evoke.

The psychoanalytic clinic testified to in these writings engages with beings infected by language through a discourse which eschews any claim to truth as constituted by evidence or to outcomes guaranteed by an invariant technique. Christian Fierens's profound examination of discourse reveals truth as founded only on a speaker's 'holding to be true,' the manner of which varies according to the discourse at play. He defines four ways, corresponding to the four discourses identified by Lacan: the university discourse holds to be true in the manner of opinion, the master's discourse in the manner of faith, the hysteric's discourse by repression and the discourse of the analyst in the manner of knowledge. This knowledge, though, is not manualisable. It is not even known. Psychoanalysis stakes itself on the gamble of an unknown knowledge coming to function in entirely singular ways that do not assemble into a universe. Moustapha Safouan, whose work and life we honour in this volume, wrote:

> You may even say [. . .] that desire is knowledge, inasmuch as it is interpretation, but it's a knowledge one is ethically required to give up, because it's also a misrecognition, insofar as any interpretation of the Other's desire makes the Other lose its authenticity, as unknown.[3]

What can be transmitted of an unknown knowledge? How to remain true to the strange, the non-family-ar? The writings herein testify to the potential for the very precision of words to surpass the familiar of anticipated meaning and surprise, survey, surge, leap *sur*, above, what we know that we know, such that something passes to us to prompt further writing and speaking, moved by a knowledge not known but activating. The attempt itself bears a remembrance of our colleague, Rod Kleiman, whose frequent flow and overflow of words made passage for a fierce love which resisted collapse into identification and honoured the authenticity of the Other as unknown.

Megan Williams

3 Safouan, M. (2204). *Four Lessons of Psychoanalysis*. A. Shane (Ed.). New York: Other Press, p. 23.

Part I

Madness

Chapter 1

Vale Rodney Kleiman (28/12/1957–23/08/2024)

David Pereira

"Life is incurable. Structure is immutable."

"Believing in Madness" is the first of Rodney Kleiman's papers to appear posthumously. As such, it is possessed of a certain aptness insofar as it forms a testament to his working life as a psychiatrist and then psychoanalyst, taking seriously the Lacanian imperative to not recede before psychosis. Rodney's work as an analyst remained driven by his firm conviction that the engagement with psychosis had much to teach us concerning the speaking being's capture within the field of language, through which it is realised that no one is immune to the effects of madness. Rodney himself revelled in the possibilities of language given through such a capture, allowing him the possibility of an acutely incisive turn of phrase born of a capacity to love madly.

His person, his presence as a fierce interlocutor, is greatly missed. His intellectual and theoretical prowess remain vigorously present for us in his writings.

DOI: 10.4324/9781003712480-2

Chapter 2

Believing in madness

Rodney Kleiman

Our reality has become virtual. So what's new? one might say.

If I had told you a year ago that an invisible substance, undetectable to the senses, a piece of dead tissue, would arrive on this planet, possibly derived from an experiment in a secret laboratory, with the capacity to infect your being, potentially to drive you to the brink of death, and that the whole world would change in unimagined ways as a consequence, you would have begun by accusing me of watching too many science fiction movies, which would be a fair criticism.

And when I persisted in saying that this is not a fantasy of mine, this is true, when I continued with absolute certainty, speaking with an unshakeable conviction, then you would have begun to doubt my sanity.

Yesterday, I was a madman; today, I am an expert, an expert prognosticator. Yesterday, I spoke delusionally, but today, I am the prescient bringer of the truth.

But the content of my speech would not have changed. I would not now be saying anything different. What has changed is that you are hearing it from a different place of knowledge, from a change, a fundamental shift in the experience of our existence. Such a knowledge makes all the difference. What you previously dismissed as paranoid ranting, as nonsense, now carries a very different significance.

Such a change in knowledge is what Jacques Lacan promoted in his approach to psychosis.[1] He suggested that we should not dismiss the content of delusional speech but attempt a different listening and, indeed, a different reading. Rather than view madness simply as a dysfunction, a deviation from sanity, to instead consider the field and function of what delusion expresses. He distinguished himself therein with this approach from Freud, who interpreted paranoia in terms of repression, of a repressed homosexuality, as he posited at the core of paranoia, which left psychosis in the same field as neurosis, undifferentiated in its mechanisms and therefore fundamentally unexplained.

1 Lacan, J. (1993). *The Psychoses: The Seminar of Jacques Lacan, 1955–56*. London: Routledge.

DOI: 10.4324/9781003712480-3

In this seminar of 1955–1956, addressed to the psychoses, Lacan, somewhat amazingly, I would note, now some 65 years ago, said the following:

> We find in the very text of the delusion a truth that isn't hidden, as it is in the neuroses, but made well and truly explicit and virtually theorised. The delusion presents it—one can't even say from the moment one has the key to it, but as soon as one takes it for what it is, a double, perfectly legible, of what is explored by theoretical investigation.[2]

It's this quotation that I continue to desire to privilege. I am convinced of its validity and, if we accept its premises, then there are consequences. Partly because I think the impact and importance of this particular form of recognition has been lost because applying this knowledge leads to a very different interpretation of the content of the psychotic phenomena. It makes of the delusion a "double" for what we, as psychoanalysts, do when we theorise. And since I don't think that all analysts are mad, contrary to popular opinion, we must conclude that theoretical thought, in the field of psychoanalysis, is the double for the apparent nonsense that delusions present to our so-called rationality. But still a non-sense which actually presents us with a truth if we read it.

"Crazy nonsense" could be, indeed is, the description given to Lacanian theorisation by many who attempt to make something from the work of Lacan and then denounce it. Let's assume they have really attempted to make something of it before denouncing it. But I'm sure he, Lacan, wasn't mad, even if he expressed, slightly flippantly on occasion perhaps, that he was psychotic. I suspect he was trying to say, in such a joke, a certain truth, that psychosis presents us with a truth that psychoanalytic theory needs to recognise and embrace as the clearest evidence and confirmation of the manner in which mankind is afflicted by the impositions of the fact that they function only through speaking, as consequence of the structural imperative of language.

God knows where the COVID-19 virus came from, let alone where it's going.

Language is a virus from outer space, William S. Burroughs wrote, saying as artists are wont to do, something touching on things they themselves don't understand.[3] Where did language come from? God knows the answer to that as well!

Language has profound effects upon our existence, perhaps even our bodily existence but unquestionably our psychic existence. In fact, language defines our existence to the extent that it is open to interpretation, given that all thought and perception exists on the basis of language and is unsupported except through words which provide the basis for all our conceptions and struggles with meaning and its limits.

2 Lacan, J. (1993). *The Psychoses*, p. 28.
3 Burroughs, W. (2014). *The Ticket That Exploded*. London: Penguin Modern Classics, p. 206.

The COVID-19 virus is a fact of science. I can speak from experience as an immune recoverer. At least I wish to believe I'm immune. But it's this other substance, language, about which madness speaks, when it warns of global disaster, of a universal affliction, of mind control or of a force conspiratorial. From the power of speech, no one is immune. No vaccine for its effects will ever arrive.

There are people around the world, in every corner of human society without exception, 1 in a 100 by all accounts, who experience this infectious language-based virus phenomenon differently. It afflicts their thoughts and their perceptions. But perceptions which we should not forget ultimately are thought. You don't need your senses, your sensorium, to perceive and receive thoughts in your head. We all hear a conversation in our heads. It's called thinking. An intact functional ego, for want of a better word, leads most of us to the delusion, a very useful delusion, that one is doing the thinking, even when the formations of the unconscious should convince one of the opposite. Because clearly, you're not in control of what you say or do despite thinking so.

The madman hears his thoughts as alien, and thus he hears the birds and the ghosts and the gods talking to him. Telepathically imposed on his consciousness as alien, foreign, not himself. He feels the approach of a dangerous, anxiety-producing presence. This external controlling influence, is it some god, some omnipotent being? Is this not a reasonable and rational question? And the answer arrives as the delusional explanation.

Perturbed by these madmen, we seek the cause of this dysfunction somewhere other than in their words and speech, when all the time, we are being told directly, by them, what ails them, because it's what ails us. It is the disease, the dis-ease of language. What ails them is what ails us all.

The delusion is the double of theoretical investigation. So the psychotic, when he speaks, is a psychoanalytic theoretician par excellence even though he might not have the first notion of or interest in psychoanalysis. This is what Lacan is telling us quite explicitly in his seminar; this is his discovery.

Now, subsequent to the *Psychoses* seminar of 1955/56, written in 1957 and first published in 1959, is his article entitled "On a question preliminary to any possible treatment of psychosis," later republished in the 1966 edition of his writings.[4] This article as published in the *Ecrits: A Selection* is introduced with the statement: "this article contains the most important parts of the seminar of 1955/56 on the psychoses."[5]

But despite that statement, you won't find the quotation from the seminar in the text of that article. It's not there. Also not there is his statement that this constitutes "the exemplary character of the field of the psychoses, and the justification for

4 Lacan, J. (1977). On a question preliminary to any possible treatment of psychosis. In: *Ecrits: A Selection*. A. Sheridan (Trans.). London: Tavistock Publications.

5 Lacan, J. (1977). On a question preliminary to any possible treatment of psychosis, p. 179.

giving it special attention."[6] Our sufficient justification might still be to learn how to read the delusion as a double of theoretical investigation.

Frankly, I think these omissions have constituted a great loss because they are, in my view, extremely important parts of the seminar on the psychoses. We have become lost in the emphasis on a cause, for example, the foreclosure of the name of the father, and later his theorisation of an unknotting of the Borromean knot constituting the subject. Now these further, different directions may well represent an advance which subverts previous renderings. But I'm leaving them aside as the initial focus for today, not because they are irrelevant—far from it—but because they are immediate distractions.

It's my view that the cogency and sheer brilliance of this initial recognition have been lost in the quest for this possible treatment, based upon the theory of causation.

Life is incurable. Structure is immutable.

I'm not saying that the locus and focus on speech should not remain at the forefront of any analytic endeavour, whatever the supposed psychic structure of the participants, however we might attempt to divide people into neurotic, perverse or psychotic individuals.

For psychoanalysis and for any understanding, however partial, of the human condition and its variety of ailments, including the particularity of each individual story, we need an approach which is based on some theorisation, at least an attempt at such.

It wasn't the headaches and fever or the swab result which convinced me I was ill with the COVID virus. It's the theory of infection, which I really have to accept. It is the capacity of humanity to recognise motive forces, which, via observation and logic, can persuade, escape sense and sensibility and confront our pride and prejudice. To accept the theory of things such as gravity, such as viral infective particles, such as atomic structure. Things that we can only know from effects. Effects which can create and destroy the whole world, which quite probably will one day.

That's what madness can tell us, the theory of psychoanalysis. I'm not pronouncing what that knowledge will do for us, what might be its utility. What we can or should do with it. We are not here to save the world, said Freud a hundred years ago. But aren't we? Now? Isn't saving the world what these times precisely confront us with? Anyway, I haven't been able to beat out of myself a possibly pointless interest in the fact that, at the least, a knowledge about what gives life meaning, however unpalatable that meaning might be to our sensibilities and however much it heightens our anxiety rather than appeases it, that this knowledge might influence people to put some more value on life, both their own life and the lives of others.

And Freud, in jokingly calling psychoanalysis a "plague," clearly didn't think it a cause unworthy of ongoing struggle.[7] Not, certainly, in order to find a vaccine

6 Lacan, J. (1977). On a question preliminary to any possible treatment of psychosis, p. 28.

7 Attributed to Freud upon his arrival with Jung to America.

for what plagues us. No doubt he was partly self-interested, to which he was surely entitled, to wish to be recognised as the discoverer of unconscious mechanisms—though the Nobel Prize committee never saw fit to recognise him in light of the potential contribution to knowledge that this work constituted. Because it's not scientific enough. It can't be proven in the laboratory.

But the madness which exists in the world, the delusions, contains definitive proof for the theory of the unconscious.

The madman wants to be believed. He is adamant that the truth, a universally important truth, has descended upon him. He's absolutely right. He doesn't doubt the validity of his experience, he doesn't doubt the importance of his knowledge. That's why he will write memoirs and treatises, like Schreber did, or endlessly champion a cause, based upon his principles, just like psychoanalysts do. Analysts are certain of one thing in the final analysis, in the finality of analysis: that they recognise in the experience of language a truth which is painful, disappointing, but still unavoidable unless you prefer to cling to illusions.

So even if it's not about a treatment, at least not for the madman, perhaps others will find benefit from the usage derived from this testimony.

Lacan calls the psychotic a "martyr of the unconscious," giving the term "martyr" its original meaning, from the Greek, which is to be a witness.[8] A martyr was a witness. That it has become a reference to religious belief, the holding of a belief, so adamantly as to be prepared to die rather than renounce this truth only further references the position of psychosis.

Lacan states that the psychotic is driven to give a testimony, an open testimony to the nature of the unconscious as consequence of language: different to the testimony of neurosis, which gives a closed testimony requiring to be deciphered.

Should we not accept this testimony of insanity about their position with respect to language, and thus the subject's relationships to language, the neurotic subject as well?

The case of Schreber and his memoirs is, for our purposes, as it was for Freud, a work in which can be read a detailed account of the psychotic's experiences, his beliefs and perceptions.[9] He derives a message for mankind from his personal story. But every psychotic is in the same position, incessantly driven to describe the relationship of man to language.

For language imposes itself upon our passive being. It persecutes us. It determines our modes of enjoyment, which are always driven by destructive drives towards death. When Schreber writes of a relationship to god, to the experiences of divine connections, via divine rays which speak, he is articulating an awareness of the experience of language and the unconscious which theorises more reliably than any psychoanalytic hypothesis.

8 Lacan, J. (1993). *The Psychoses*, p. 132.

9 Freud, S. (2011). Psychoanalytic notes on an autobiographical account of a case of paranoia. SE 12: 9–82.

When the birds speak, when the divine rays connect him to god, when he ponders what it is like to be a woman enjoying sexual intercourse, he poses an answer to the questions which are the province of psychoanalytic theorists par excellence. It's a conspiracy theory which is actually true.

The delusion presents a message on the nature of neurosis. They know not what they say. That is what gives what they say its worth. Something to be read. Different but analogous to the neurotic, who also doesn't know what they are saying but can't stop repeating themselves in the endeavour, presenting something therein to be deciphered.

Language is a virus. Not derived from outer space, nor from nonexistent deities, but from the internalised, alienating fact of others, threatening others, hellish others, essential others, themselves caught in the web of mortal suffering, mutilating, cohabitating, isolating together. Which never stops the spread. It has invaded our minds and our bodies. It is unnatural.

This truth is what madness attests—sufficient justification to convince us to listen to the cruel truth contained in the testimony of madness.

Why does this happen? Why does the psychotic speak this truth that constitutes a theory of language and man's relation to language? There dawns on him the realisation that something is very amiss with the world and with the way people are relating to each other, and he finds himself overcome with the difficulty of not experiencing an overwhelming angst coupled with an untold suffering that his "living" produces and encompasses. And then he finds an answer. The delusion contains the answer to this terrifying and terrible state of being. He doesn't just breathe its last statement, final dying words, "the horror! the horror!" the darkness at the heart of man's journey.[10]

The delusion writes a story that speaks of universal suffering, whilst the neurotic is absorbed in explaining his own particular sad tale of woe. The psychotic is sharing with us the true version of the origin of universal suffering, which leaves us in a very different place when confronted by their words. How to respond to a universal version of what troubles them? What about them as an individual, as opposed to simply a messenger of the truth?

That's a dilemma to return us to a place even prior to the preliminary questioning of any possible treatment of psychosis.

10 Conrad, J. (1902). *Heart of Darkness*. London: Blackwood and Sons, p. 63.

Chapter 3

Believing in Ondine

Debbie Plastow

Introduction

In his *R.S.I.* seminar of 1974–1975,[1] Lacan cites a theatrical work by Giraudoux, asserting:

> What is striking in the symptom, in this something that smooches [*se bécote*] with the unconscious, is that one *believes it* [*y croit*]. There are so few sexual relations that I recommend for that the reading of something which is a very beautiful novel *Ondine*.[2] *Ondine* manifests what is in question [. . .][3]

Lacan's statement is notable not only for his high praise of this work of Giraudoux but also for its intriguing proposition that *Ondine* manifests what is in question. What is it in Giraudoux's tale that Lacan is alluding to here, and how might we consider this in relation to the symptom? In this chapter, I would like to interrogate the way in which Lacan takes up particular aspects of *Ondine* in the seminar of 21**st** January 1975 in his conceptualisation of neurosis and psychosis. I would specifically like to put into question the use of the adverbial phrase "*y croire*" ("to believe it" or literally, "*to believe there*" *in Lacan's French*) and to elaborate upon this. This critical phrase comes to signify something that is lost in Cormac Gallagher's translation; therefore, a more literal translation of the French version of the seminar will be utilised in this chapter.[4] I will propose that "to believe it" is an unmediated relation, which is a symptom of or a manifestation of something that might lead to psychosis.

1 Lacan, J. (1974–1975a). *R.S.I. Séminaire 1974–1975*. Paris: Editions de l'Association Freudienne Internationale. Publication hors commerce.
2 Giraudoux, J. (2016 [1939]). *Ondine. Intermezzo*. [Présentation par Hélène Laplace-Claverie]. Paris: Flammarion.
3 Lacan, J. (1974–1975a). *R.S.I. Séminaire 1974–1975*, session of 21.1.1975, p. 65. [My trans. and emphasis].
4 Thanks are extended to Michael Gerard Plastow for assisting with translations of Lacan's seminar for this chapter.

DOI: 10.4324/9781003712480-4

Ondine

Jean Giraudoux's fantastical story was inspired by a fairy tale titled *Undine,* penned in 1811 by Count Frédérik de La Motte-Fouqué. Giraudoux adapted this tale to create *Ondine*, a play in three acts that was published in 1939.

Central to Giraudoux's tale are a fisherman named Auguste and his wife, Eugénie. Act One opens with an intense discussion between Auguste and Eugénie in their cottage during a violent thunderstorm. Auguste is despairing over the whereabouts and wild, erratic behaviour of their daughter, Ondine, whom Eugénie believes she can hear singing in the middle of the lake.

An undine or ondine is "a female water-sprite" or "nymph,"[5] one of the four spirits of nature, along with the "sylph," a being which inhabits the air, "salamander," which lives in fire, and "gnome,"[6] fabled to inhabit the earth and guard its treasures. From Latin, "*unde*" denotes "from where or whence," and describes a *movement*, specifically an undulation or "wave." Thus we propose here that an undine is not a graspable object or something that might be pinned down but a movement, something elusive, always slipping away, constantly disappearing and reappearing at whim.

In the second scene, a stranger, Le Chevalier, unexpectedly arrives at the family's home, seeking refuge from the storm. The stranger presents himself as Ritter Hans von Wittenstein zu Wittenstein and proceeds to take advantage of his hosts' humble hospitality by inviting himself to a dinner of blue trout whilst detailing feats exemplifying his prowess and courage. He speaks of the innumerable perfections of his fiancée, Countess Bertha, whom he is planning to impress with tales of his daring adventures.

In the third scene, we are just as suddenly confronted by Ondine, who bursts in and immediately seizes the opportunity to seduce the guest with words of flattery uttered in a provocative and flirtatious manner. Ondine's first words, "How handsome you are!"[7] have the desired effect on Le Chevalier, and her parents' attempts to send her to her room prove futile. Le Chevalier, stunned and bewitched, even when Ondine throws his blue trout out of the window and back into the lake, falls in love with her. Unable to resist Ondine's charms, by the seventh scene, over a glass or two of Moselle, Le Chevalier seeks Auguste and Eugénie's consent for their daughter's hand in marriage.

The old fisherman, however, attempts to dissuade Hans from this impulsive idea, revealing that Ondine is not, in fact, their daughter but a child of nature whom

5 In *R.S.I.*, Lacan uses the word "ondine," which corresponds with the title of Giraudoux's play. In Gallagher's translation of the seminar, the word "ondine" is replaced with "water sprite." The word "ondine" is therefore used in this chapter as a literal translation of Lacan's words from the French version of his seminar.

6 O.E.D. (1973 [1932]). *Shorter Oxford English Dictionary on Historical Principles*. 3rd Edition. Oxford: Clarendon Press, p. 2413.

7 Giraudoux, J. (2016 [1939]). *Ondine. Intermezzo*, p. 169. [My trans.].

they adopted after they discovered her as an infant abandoned on the shore of the lake. Auguste speaks of Ondine as a phenomenon, frequently disappearing without a trace and returning at will, declaring: "Ondine, that's a dream! There is no Ondine."[8] Anguished, he pleads with his wife, "You, you believe *it* [*y croit*], you believe *in* [à] Ondine, Eugénie?"[9]

It is these words from Giraudoux's play that Lacan takes up in the *R.S.I.* seminar, giving us a glimpse into Lacan's well-known proposition that there is no sexual relation. In Lacan's introductory remarks leading to his reference to *Ondine,* he states, "*The woman* [*La femme*] does not ek-sist. [. . .] to say *The woman,* is not the same thing as to say *women* [*les femmes*]."[10] Lacan's distinction between "*The* woman" and "women" is crucial to his theorisation of woman as symptom.

In Gallagher's translation of Lacan's subsequent statement, we read, "What is striking in the symptom, in this something which gives *a little peck* to the unconscious, is that *it* is believed."[11] However, a more literal translation might be: "What is striking in the symptom, in this something that *smooches* [*se bécote*] with the unconscious, is that one believes *it* [*y croit*]."[12]

These two contrasting translations provide an initial glimpse at what might be in question here. Gallagher's "little peck" sounds prudish in comparison to something that "smooches" with the unconscious. Moreover, a peck—translated by Gallagher as a noun—denotes something transitory yet fixed, whereas the intransitive verb "smooches" conveys a sense of movement, an undulating movement perhaps. Moreover, like the elusive ondine, something that smooches with the unconscious denotes something fluid that cannot easily be grasped or pinned down but constantly slips away.

Also central to Lacan's theorisation here is the French pronoun "*y*," which is uttered by Auguste in his impassioned plea to Eugénie: "[. . .] you believe *it* [*y croit*] [. . .]."[13] We note that the object pronoun "it" is placed in the position of subject in Gallagher's translation: "[. . .] *it* is believed." However, the word "*y*" is an adverbial pronoun that functions to replace the noun representing place, that is, the "where" or "there" of the utterance. Lacan takes up the tale of *Ondine* to elaborate this. He states:

> [. . .] A woman in the life of a man is something he believes *in* [*à croire*], he believes that there is one, sometimes two or three, and what moreover is interesting here is that he can only believe in one. He believes [*il croit*] that there

8 Giraudoux, J. (2016 [1939]). *Ondine. Intermezzo*, p. 188. [My trans.].
9 Giraudoux, J. (2016 [1939]). *Ondine. Intermezzo*, p. 188. [My trans. and emphasis].
10 Lacan, J. (1974–1975a). *R.S.I. Séminaire 1974–1975*, session of 21.1.75, p. 64. [My trans. and emphasis].
11 Lacan, J. (1974–1975b). Seminar of R.S.I. 1994–1975. C. Gallagher (Trans.). Session of 21.1.75, p. 63. http://www.lacaninireland.com. [My emphasis].
12 Lacan, J. (1974–1975a). *R.S.I. Séminaire 1974–1975*, session of 21.1.75, p. 65. [My trans. and emphasis].
13 Giraudoux, J. (2016 [1939]). *Ondine. Intermezzo*, p. 188. [My trans. and emphasis].

> is a species, in the style of sylphs or ondines. What is it to believe in sylphs or ondines? I point out to you that one says believe *in* [*croire à*] in this case. And even that the French tongue adds to it this reinforcement of what is not believe *in*, but believe *it* [*croire y*], believe *there* [*croire là*].[14]

Here Lacan contrasts "to believe *in* [it]" [*croire à*], in which there is an indirect object, with "to believe *it*" or "to believe *there*" [*y croire* or *croire là*], in which there is a direct object. Thus, "to believe *in* it" or "to believe *in* her" constitutes a mediated relation to the object. On the other hand, "to believe *it*" or the more literal "to believe *there*" is an unmediated relation that conveys the sense of something fixed, such as that which might be heard in psychosis. Gallagher's translation, "[. . .] *it* is believed," also evokes fixity, with something being pinned down. Schreber does not believe *in* God; he believes *it*, he believes God, he believes *them*, the voices.

This question of whether one might "believe *in* it" or "believe *it*" is central to the story of *Ondine.* We discover that for Auguste, *The* Ondine does not exist. He does not believe *it.* He declares to Eugénie and Le Chevalier, "Ondine, that's a dream! There's no Ondine." From this impassioned plea, we ascertain that for Auguste, she is *an* ondine, that is, one of many ondines. Moreover, Ondine also considers herself as being just one of a number of ondines, and this is reflected in her words when introducing herself. When the queen, Yseult, summons her, Ondine responds in the following manner:

Yseult: Do you want my advice, dear little Ondine?
Ondine: Yes, I am an ondine.
Yseult: You can listen to me, you are fifteen years old.
Ondine: Fifteen years in a month. And I was born centuries ago and I will never die.[15]

Ondine recites these same lines on each occasion that she introduces herself. Her statement, "I am *an* ondine," repeated at various points in the tale, informs us that from Ondine's point of view, she is not "*The* Ondine" but one of a species. She is one of any number of ondines; sometimes in the story there are two others or even three. The other ondines appear at inopportune moments, such as when she is alone with Le Chevalier. They attempt to put an end to his infatuation with Ondine, using their wit and charms to try to seduce and distract him, for they know that if Ondine marries him, she is destined to become mortal, thereby losing her mythical status as *an* ondine.

Let us return to the desperate interchange between Auguste and his wife in the presence of Le Chevalier. Auguste is pleading with Eugénie in an attempt to

14 Lacan, J. (1974–1975a). *R.S.I. Séminaire 1974–1975*, session of 21.1.75, pp. 65–66. [My trans. and emphasis].
15 Giraudoux, J. (2016 [1939]). *Ondine. Intermezzo*, p. 240. [My trans.].

convince her that Ondine is a dream. He asks her, "Do you believe *it*?" [*y crois*]. Eugénie retorts, "I believe [*je crois*] that you are going a bit mad, my poor Auguste." She turns to Le Chevalier, explaining, "It's his Moselle. It's treacherous. It's like his history of *paillettes*."[16]

These *paillettes*, the sequins, sparkly specks, or the starry-eyed story or account, are something one might only catch a glimpse of. Here, Eugénie's glittery and seemingly sympathetic response to her husband's question is evasive, avoiding his question. Auguste's worst fear is realised. His wife does not believe *in* it, but she believes *it* [*y croit*], that there is just one, *The* one and only Ondine. And we are aware that believing *it* corresponds with Lacan's notion of the psychotic believing *it* or believing *them,* believing *the voices*. We note here that Le Chevalier is also starry-eyed and dazzled by Ondine, but in his blinded state of being in love.

So how can we conceptualise psychosis as opposed to the madness of being in love? Here, Lacan again makes reference to *Ondine*, speaking of the state of being *in love* as a mediated relation:

> [I]t is the major love, it is the one that is founded on the following: that one believes *her* [*la croit*], that one believes *her* [*la croit*] because one has never had proof that she might not be absolutely authentic. But this believing *her* [*la croire*] is nonetheless this something upon which one becomes completely blind, which serves as a *plug*, if I might say so, it's what I already said, to believe *it* [*y croire*], which is a thing that can be very seriously put into question.[17]

Lacan thus speaks of the blindness of being in love. To believe *her*, or to be *in* love with her, leads one to become "completely blind." However, this state of being in love is not equivalent to simply believing *her* or believing *it* but believing *in* her, which constitutes a mediated relation.

Here, we are reminded of Lacan's remarkable statement: "I love you, but, because inexplicably I love *in* you something more than you—the object petit *a*—I mutilate you."[18] Could such a mediated relation serve as a plug for the "believing *it*" or "believing *there*" of psychosis? Lacan again refers to *Ondine* to elaborate something of this:

> [T]o believe that there is one of them, God knows where that takes you, that takes you up to the point of believing that there is *The [La], The [La]* which is a quite fallacious belief. Nobody says *the* sylph, or *the* ondine, there is *an* ondine

16 Giraudoux, J. (2016 [1939]). *Ondine. Intermezzo*, p. 189.

17 Lacan, J. (1974–1975a). *R.S.I. Séminaire 1974–1975*, session of 21.1.75, pp. 66–67. [My trans. and emphasis].

18 Lacan, J. (1977). *The Four Fundamental Concepts of Psycho-Analysis*. J-A. Miller (Ed.), A. Sheridan (Trans.). New York & London: W. W. Norton & Co, session of 24.6.1964, p. 263. [My emphasis].

> or *a* sylph. There is a spirit, there are spirits for certain people. But all of that only ever makes a plural. It is a question of knowing what is the sense of that. What sense that to believe *it* [*y croire*] has and if there is not something quite necessitated in the fact that, to believe *it* [*y croire*], there is no better means than *la croire*, to believe her.[19]

Such a differentiation made by Lacan provides a sparkly glimpse of how neurosis and psychosis might be manifested. In psychosis, as Lacan proposes here, one "believes *it*" or "believes *there*," that there is *The* Ondine. However, in order to believe *her*, one must also believe *in* her, one believes *in* what she says. Thus, "to believe *in* her" [*la croire*], constitutes the mediated relation, providing a plug for the unmediated "to believe *there*" or "to believe *it*" [*y croire*] of psychosis. Lacan continues:

> This is what makes a difference between neurosis and psychosis. In psychosis, everything is there, the voices [*les voix*], they believe *it* [*ils y croient*]. Not only do they believe *it* [*ils y croient*] but they believe *them* [*ils les croient*]. And yet everything is there, in this limit.[20]

Here, Lacan takes the unmediated "believing it" or "believing there" one step further, to its limit. This fixed "limit" or endpoint in which "everything is there" manifests psychosis. The psychotic believes *it*, he believes *them*, he believes the voices.

However, Lacan goes on to state that

> Believing her [*la croire*] is, thank God, a widespread condition because, all the same, it provides company, you are no longer all alone. And that is why love is precious, eh!, rarely realised, as everyone knows only lasting for a time and all the same made up of the fact that it is essentially this split or crack in the wall [*cette fracture du mur*] where one can only give oneself a bump on the forehead, in short, that is what is in question.[21]

In speaking of "believing her" [*la croire*] as "a widespread condition," Lacan is referring to the state of being in love. Moreover, Lacan proposes that a woman is a symptom to a man. Implicit in the phrase "believing her" is the mediating "in," that is, one "believes *in* her," one believes *in* her as his symptom.

We note that when Lacan speaks of "*this split* or *crack* in the wall," he uses a noun rather than a verb, although in Gallagher's translation, it is an action, a

19 Lacan, J. (1974–1975a). *R.S.I. Séminaire 1974–1975*, session of 21.1.75, p. 67. [My trans. and emphasis].
20 Lacan, J. (1974–1975a). *R.S.I. Séminaire 1974–1975*, p. 66. [My trans. and emphasis].
21 Lacan, J. (1974–1975a). *R.S.I. Séminaire 1974–1975*, p. 66. [My trans.].

"*breaking down of* the wall".[22] Through this split in the wall, the wall—or the real—might be considered a crack through which we could glimpse something, perhaps a few *paillettes*, some specks or sparkly things.

Conclusion

The beauty of the tale of *Ondine* is that there is no singular ondine. If *The* woman or *The* Ondine does not exist, then to believe *it* or to believe *there*, to believe in the singular, is an unmediated relation. A belief in a sexual relation is something that approaches psychosis, as President Schreber demonstrates. Lacan's notable statement, "I love you, but, because inexplicably I love *in* you something more than you [. . .]" gives us a glimpse of something sparkly that might equate to the madness of being *in* love, inevitably resulting in a bump on the head. However, this mediated relation, "to love *in* you," "to believe *in* her," or, moreover, "to believe *in* it," allows one the possibility of believing *in* a symptom. To believe *in* it, to believe in a symptom, this something that smooches with the unconscious, opens up an opportunity for movement, an undulating movement perhaps, something that might be worked in an analysis or through writing.

22 Lacan, J. (1974–1975b). Seminar of R.S.I. 1994–1975, session of 21.1.75, p. 64.

Chapter 4

The madness of the analyst

Peter Gunn

At the invitation of his friend, the psychiatrist Henri Ey, in 1946, Lacan gave the opening presentation at a conference at the Bonneval Psychiatric Hospital in northern France. The original title of the conference made it appear rather academic and lifeless: "The Problem of the Psychogenesis of the Neuroses and the Psychoses."

Lacan, on the other hand, entitled his paper, "Remarks on Psychic Causality" and with that cut both to the chase and to the cause. No longer confined to the phenomenology of mental illness, psychic causality is now taken as *structural*: it is indigenous to the human psyche, in becoming. That is, the cause is now alive. As such, however, it is now also unfathomable and can be thought only as madness.

Here is Lacan from the published version of his paper:

> [I]n consigning the causality of [this] madness to the unfathomable decision whereby the human being [. . .] misrecognises his liberation, in the snare of fate that deceives them about a freedom they have not in the least conquered, I am merely restating the ancient formula of the Ancients.[1]

And if Lacan would appear here to be deferring to the wisdom of the ancients, he doesn't just meekly restate this ancient formula. He *rewrites* it, perhaps on the blackboard, in its original language, Ancient Greek: Γένοἰ οἷος έσςὶ [*Genoio hoios essi*]. Furthermore, even with this rewriting, Lacan goes further. Much like Nietzsche in *The Gay Science*, in appropriating this line of Pindar, the Greek lyric poet of the fifth century BC, Lacan once again cuts: He leaves out the last word.[2]

That last word is μαθών [*mathon*], which in this context can be taken to mean "measure" or "learning." If we retain that word, this formula might be rendered as "Become who you are in good measure" or "Become who you are by learning."

1 Lacan, J. (2006 [1946]). Presentation on Psychical Causality. In: *Écrits*. Bruce Fink (Trans.). New York: W. W. Norton & Company, pp. 143–144 [translation modified].

2 See Babich, B. E. (2003). Nietzsche's imperative as a friend's encomium: On becoming the one you are, ethics, and blessing. In: *Nietzsche-Studien*, vol. 33, pp. 30–31.

DOI: 10.4324/9781003712480-5

And whilst such an incitement to self-improvement might be well received in some quarters, it is also one which is well worn.

With Lacan's elision, what was advice becomes apophthegm. That is, from the Greek, it becomes itself a speaking out. Whereas μαθών [*mathon*] acts to qualify, or put conditions on, the urgency of speaking. Without that word, the formula must be rendered as direct discourse. It has the liveliness of an address, in the imperative: "Become who you are!"

At the same time, however, by writing in Greek and, in addition, using all the diacritics which indicate the quality of the breath to be used in pronunciation, Lacan draws our attention to what is betrayed by any such address.

What Lacan's rewriting shows, at least on my reading, is that when taken to the level of the letter, this address, and, indeed, any saying, any act of speaking, carries a force akin to that of black letter law. But this force is radically foreign, including to the speaker. It owes its authority neither to precedent nor, indeed, to rhetoric. Nor can it be remedied, whether by learning or some other prescription.

For this reason, this force can only be thought of as madness. Looked at another way, however, this madness is itself an opening, one which is knotted to becoming, becoming who you are, as human.

❦ ❦ ❦

In 1958, 12 years after "Remarks on Psychic Causality," Lacan returns to this speaking-madness in his paper "On a Question Preliminary to Any Possible Treatment of Psychosis." This is despite the fact that he is, at least ostensibly, discussing the case of someone who would usually be thought to most clearly satisfy the criteria for sequestration: Judge Daniel Paul Schreber.

Schreber's own writing, in the form of his book, *Memoirs of My Mental Illness*, was closely read by both Freud and Lacan. Lacan drew on it extensively during *The Psychoses*, his seminar of 1955 to '56. But he did so not so much by way of elucidating psychosis but of elucidating the structure of the subject itself.

Here is Lacan on madness from his 1958 paper:

> What I am asserting here is that, in recognizing the drama of madness, reason is doing what it likes best, *sua res agitur* [that is, it *concerns you*], because it is in man's relation to the signifier that this drama is situated.
>
> The danger people mention of becoming as mad as the patient no more intimidates me than it did Freud.
>
> Like Freud, I hold that we must listen to the speaker, when what is at stake is a message that does not come from a subject beyond language, but from speech beyond the subject. [. . .]
>
> Here we encounter anew [. . .] what I said in my dialogue with Henri Ey [Lacan quotes himself]: "And as for the being of man, not only can it not be

understood without madness, but it would not be the being of man if it did not carry madness within itself as the limit of his freedom."[3]

Notwithstanding Lacan's disavowal of being intimidated by the risk of going mad, this madness is one which we must place on the side of the analyst. If, as Lacan expressed it in 1946, the being of man cannot be understood without madness, this implies that in listening, the analyst must take difference to the point of madness.

I am reminded here of something Lacan says in his *Note Italienne* concerning the end of the analysis, in this case, the end of the analysis of the becoming-analyst: "Thenceforth he knows being reject. This is what [his] analyst must have at least made him feel. If he is not carried by it to enthusiasm, he may well have had an analysis, but of analyst no chance."[4]

Now we know, if only from the Greek etymology of the word, how close enthusiasm is to madness. But this madness cannot be sequestered, not even within the parameters of what might be considered proper to the formation of the analyst.

This recalls another formula, *Wo Es War, Soll Ich Werden*. Freud's maxim for the practice of psychoanalysis. It can be translated into English as *There Where It Was, There Must I Become*. But such a definitive reference to "It" carries with it a tendency to personification. The effect is to keep saying bound to the safety of the already-said, that is, to what It, taken to be Someone, has prescribed.

In order to cut this bigwig down to size, rather than translating Freud's German into its standard French equivalent, Lacan once again rewrites it, but in his *lalangue*.[5] That is to say, he rewrites it in terms of enjoyment, the enjoyment of what might be heard when he, in particular, speaks.

Lacan does this in his 1956 paper, "The Freudian Thing."[6] Taking advantage of the homophony, in French, between "*Là où c'était*" and "*Là où s'était,*" Lacan writes, "There where it was [*Là où c'était*]" as "There where it was itself [*là où s'était*]."

What is enjoined with Freud's maxim is then, necessarily, also transformed. It becomes "There where it was itself [*là où s'était*], it is my task to come toward being [*c'est mon devoir que je vienne à être*]."

3 Lacan, J. (2006 [1958]). On a question prior to any possible treatment of psychosis. In: *Écrits*. Bruce Fink (Trans.). New York: W. W. Norton & Company, pp. 478–479.

4 Lacan, J. (2001 [1973]). Note italienne. In: *Autres Écrits*. Paris: Éditions du Seuil, p. 309 [my trans.].

5 In using "*lalangue*" here, I am anticipating the first occasion on which Lacan writes this neologism. In the first lesson of his seminar *The Knowledge of the Psychoanalyst*, he indicates that *lalangue* is, in effect, the writing which insists in slips of the tongue (see Lacan, J. (2013 [1971]), p. 23). Indeed, three years later, in "La troisième," Lacan will explicitly re-define the unconscious itself in terms of *lalangue*. He speaks there of it being made of the enjoyment of speaking: "The subject-supposed-to-know, which is the analyst in the transference, is not incorrectly supposed if he knows that the unconscious consists of being a knowledge which is articulated by *lalangue*. The body which speaks it is only knotted to it by the real from which it enjoys itself."

6 Lacan, J. (2006 [1956]). The Freudian thing or the meaning of the return to Freud in psychoanalysis. In: *Écrits*. Bruce Fink (Trans.). New York: W. W. Norton & Company, pp. 334–363.

Passing in this way from the prescriptions of the said to the exigencies of saying, Freud's aphorism can be read as specifying the strangeness of the psychoanalytic project itself. This is that strangeness which is intrinsic to the act of speaking as such, inasmuch as in that act, there is enjoyment, but an enjoyment which is utterly eccentric to our being. To put this more intimately, taking advantage of another Lacanian invention, we can say that for psychoanalysis the *parlêtre*, the *speak-being*, is *always-about-to-come*, but from elsewhere.[7]

❦ ❦ ❦

Speaking of direct address, let me come now to another writing, that of Marguerite Duras.

Sometime in the mid-1960s, Lacan asked to meet with Duras. According to Duras, he did so in order to talk about *The Ravishing of Lol V. Stein*, her recently published novel. It seems that for Lacan, this novel was exemplary, not so much as a novel but as a case study. According to Duras, "[Lacan] told [her] that it was a clinically perfect delirium."[8]

As Duras tells it, they met in a Parisian bistro at midnight. As the French psychoanalyst Jean Allouch tells it, this meeting has all the romance of an incident in a spy novel or, more to the point, in an affair.[9]

But if, at the outset of this affair, Lacan positioned himself as the seducer, his opening gambit could hardly be said to have been seductive. Even as he approached Duras, still threading his way between the empty tables, he felt obliged to cry out, "You don't know what you're saying."[10]

7 Again, in using *parlêtre* here, I am anticipating Lacan's first writing of this neologism, in this case in a paper which was itself a re-writing. In 1975, at the Sorbonne in Paris, Lacan gave the opening address of The Fifth James Joyce International Forum. He later produced a much-revised written version of his presentation. This was eventually published in the volume *Joyce & Paris*, with the title "Joyce le Symptôme." Lacan, J. (1979 [1975]). *Joyce & Paris 1902 . . . 1920–1940 . . . 1975: Papers from the Fifth International James Joyce Symposium*. Paris 16–20 June 1975, Presses universitaires de Lille/Éditions du CNRS, Lille, 1979, pp. 59–94; https://www.freud2lacan.com/docs/Joyce-le-Symptôme-2-3col.pdf, viewed October 2020. It was later included in the anthology *Autres écrits*, using the same title. To distinguish it from Eric Laurent's transcription of Lacan's presentation, this text has, however, come to be referred to as "Joyce le Symptôme II" (see Price, A. 2014, "In the Nebohood of Joyce and Lacan," LCExpress, 2, 14, pp. 1–24). Crucially, in proposing there that his parlêtre might supersede Freud's unconscious, Lacan comments that "the fact that man makes a living of being" [*le fait qu'il vit de l'être*] necessitates that he makes a void of it [*qu'il vide l'être*]. In saying this, he plays on the homophony in French between "vit" and "vide." This (*ça*) unconscious must, therefore, be read [*inconscient, qu'on lit ça*].

8 Duras, M. (1970 [1969]). An interview with Marguerite Duras by Jacques Rivette and Jean Narboni. In: *Destroy She Said*, B. Bray and H. L. Cumberford (Trans.). New York: Grove Press, p. 129.

9 Allouch, J. (2009). *Les impromptus de Lacan: 543 bons mots recueillis par Jean Allouch*. Paris: Fayard, p. 242.

10 Allouch, J. (2009). *Les impromptus de Lacan*, p. 242.

If Lacan set up the meeting, it would be a sleight of hand to position him as the *auteur* of this *mise en scène*. Nor do I think that we should identify him as playing the part of the great psychoanalyst, one who is in a position to make a rather backhanded acknowledgement of the workings of an interlocutor's unconscious.

Lacan is not being stand-offish here; on the contrary, he himself is implicated.

I am guided here by something Lacan himself says. In his 1965 article "Homage to Marguerite Duras, on *Le ravissement de Lol V. Stein*," Lacan draws on his own polyphonic and polymorphous associations to that name. Finding a coded reference to the guessing game Paper, Scissors, Stone, he is led to observe that "in the game of death [*au jeu de la mourre*] you lose yourself."[11]

And already, just in reading this in French, we might ourselves get a little lost. The phrase which Lacan uses, which I've translated as "the game of death," is *au jeu de la mourre*. In saying this out loud, those who are French speakers will no doubt hear the equivocation. As written, *la mourre* means death, but as read, and thus also sounded, it means love (*l'amour*). So perhaps we should rather say, "in the game of love/death you lose yourself."

But if Lacan wasn't the architect of this affair, who was? Was it, in fact, Duras? Or was it someone or something else?

Whoever or whatever it was, I now want to leave to one side any consideration of either of these individuals, Lacan and Duras, in terms of, say, their motivation. What I am interested in, rather, is the architecture. That is, what I am interested in is the *structure* of this imbroglio.

What might give us a clue here is Duras, not Duras the individual but her *writing*, in the particularity of its style, what some French scholars call *l'écriture durassienne*.[12] Let us consider, from this perspective, *La maladie de la mort* [*The Malady of Death*].[13]

This "novel," if, indeed, it can be regarded as a novel, or, indeed, any other literary genre, was published 18 years after *Le ravissement de Lol V.* Stein. It consists of a series of exchanges between two unnamed characters. The exchanges are given only at third hand, by way of reported speech. There is a "You," who, for reasons which are already all too evident, we take to be a man, and a "She" or a "Her," who might be a prostitute and who, since she is referred to only by feminine pronouns, and otherwise only by way of what is *not* there, we take to be a woman.

Here is how *The Malady of Death* sets the scene:

> You wouldn't have known her, you'd have seen her everywhere at once, in a hotel, in a street, in a book, in a film, in yourself, your inmost self, when your

11 Lacan, J. (1965). Hommage fait a Marguerite Duras, du ravissement de Lol V. Stein. In: *Cahiers Renaud-Barrault*. Paris: Gallimard, p. 52. https://www.freud2lacan.com/docs/Lacan-bilingual-Homage_Duras.pdf, viewed October 2020 [my trans.].

12 See for example, Ledwina, A. (2011). L'écriture durassienne—mise en scène de l'ellipse et de l'innommable. In: *Synergies Pologne*, vol. 8, pp. 21–28.

13 Duras, M. (1986 [1982]). *The Malady of Death*. B. Bray (Trans.). New York: Grove Press.

> sex grew erect in the night, seeking somewhere to put itself, somewhere to shed its load of tears.[14]

Then, towards the end of the book, we come upon the following:

> You ask how the sentiment of love could arise. She answers you. Perhaps from a sudden lapse in the logic of the universe. She says: For example, through a mistake.[15]

"You" continues:

> Could the sentiment of love arise from other things? You beg her to say. She says: From everything, from the flight of a night bird, from sleep [. . .] She says: Look. She opens her legs and in the hollow of her spreading legs you see the dark night at last. You say: It was there, the dark night. It's there.[16]

Are we aroused by the madness of these words? More fool us. So enlivened, we might now take the *more* of "more to the point," the phrase which I used just now, to point to us. And if this is the opening of love, it is a love which opens *us* onto death.

What we encounter in Duras's love-death-writing is *more*, that is, the excess of the word when spoken. It is to this unfathomable *more* that I take Lacan to be referring when, in 1976, in the seminar on Joyce, he speaks of the parasitic real of *jouissance*.[17]

But if we, speakers of standard English, spell *more* as "more," some might hear another equivocation here. As sounded, in standard English, "maw" is the throat, especially of some voracious animal. But for those exposed to the patois of the Scottish Lowlands, whether directly through their mother tongue or indirectly through its infiltration into American popular culture by way of Appalachian song, it can also be heard as "maw," that is, "mother."[18] With this rewriting, *more* becomes the voracious and also prohibited Mother of fact and fable.

Something similar seems to have happened for Lacan in his seminar on Joyce with his own word, *jouissance*. Hearing *jouissance* homophonically, by way of his own *lalangue*, he is led once again to rewrite it. The result this time is an indecipherable holophrase: *j'ouïs-sens*.[19] In being read, however, this holophrase can be

14 Duras, M. (1986 [1982]). *The Malady of Death*, p. 1.
15 Duras, M. (1986 [1982]). *The Malady of Death*, p. 50.
16 Duras, M. (1986 [1982]). *The Malady of Death*, p. 51.
17 Lacan, J. (2016 [1976]). *The Sinthome, the Seminar of Jacques Lacan Book XXIII*. J.-A. Miller (Ed.), A. R. Price (Trans.). Cambridge: Polity, session of 13.1.76, p. 58.
18 See for example, Ritchie, F. and Orr, D. (2014). *Wayfaring Strangers, the Musical Voyage from Scotland and Ulster to Appalachia*. Chapel Hill: University of North Carolina.
19 Lacan, J. (2013 [1976]). *The Sinthome, the Seminar of Jacques Lacan Book XXIII*, p. 58.

rendered, in French, as, *j'ouïs sens*. This can in turn be translated into English as, "I hear sense."

What does this tell us? It tells us that in listening with Freud's suspended attention, we must listen, first of all and paradoxically, by *seeing*. This is what is required if we are to follow Lacan's call to take speech to the letter. It is only by *seeing* speech, seeing it as we hear it, as writing, that we are in a position to keep attending to what Lacan refers to in 1958, in his paper "On a Question Preliminary to Any Possible Treatment of Psychosis," as "speech beyond the subject."[20]

Taking this to heart, rather than being a teaching, even a teaching concerning the unconscious, Lacan's cry, "You don't know what you're saying," must first of all be taken as a writing. It is a writing of the not-known by which the unconscious enacts itself. As a consequence, I propose that prior to any meaning which we might ascribe to these words and to any knowledge we might ascribe to whoever it is who is speaking them, this cry gives voice.

Personified by the anonymous *She*, what *l'écriture durassienne* opens on to then is something which, though otherwise nothing, very clearly implicates us: a sudden lapse in the logic of the universe. In a word, it opens onto death.

But just because it is *une écriture*, the writing of a certain *lalangue*, the nothing of death is in this way entangled with and spliced to love. This, in any event, is how I now understand what Lacan says in his seminar *Le Sinthome* when, at the same time as he writes that holophrase *j'ouïs-sens*, he makes mention of a different order of teaching: "we teach the analysand to splice, to perform a splice, between his *sinthome* and the parasitic real of *jouissance*."[21] In re-reading this, I recall that, three years earlier, in his seminar *Encore*, Lacan had said of love that it makes up for or, alternatively, makes do with (*supplée au*) the absence or failure of the sexual relation.[22]

❦ ❦ ❦

Following this reference by Lacan to the responsibility of the analyst, and to conclude, I would like to give a brief clinical illustration of this coincidence of failure, death and love. The clinic I have in mind is that of someone who was an almost exact contemporary of Lacan, the English psychoanalyst Margaret Little.

Little was at a loss to know how to gain any purchase on the extreme distress of one of her analysands, whom she calls Frieda, following the sudden death of an old

20 Lacan, J. (2006 [1958]). On a question prior to any possible treatment of psychosis, p. 479.
21 Lacan, J. (2016 [1976]). *The Sinthome, the Seminar of Jacques Lacan Book XXIII*, p. 58.
22 Lacan, J. (1998 [1973]). *On Feminine Sexuality, The Limits of Love and Knowledge, Book XX Encore 1972–1973*. J.-A. Miller (Ed.), B. Fink (Trans.). New York: W. W. Norton, p. 45 (session of 16.1.73).

family friend, who she calls Ilse. Such was this distress that Frieda began to almost hallucinate her friend:

> [Frieda] saw Ilse in buses, in the street, in shops, ran after her, only to find it was someone else. My interpretations that she wanted me magically to bring Ilse to life again and that she wanted to punish herself and her environment for her unhappiness, fell on deaf ears; nothing reached her. She could not lie down; she sat for a few minutes at a time and ranged round the room, weeping and wringing her hands.[23]

Pushed to the limit, both by Frieda's resistance to her many, well-considered interpretations but also by the life-threatening immediacy of Frieda's distress, Little comes to life as an analyst. She takes the risk of speaking of her own difficulty in being present to her analysand's distress. In doing so, it becomes clear that she ended up putting herself right there, in the middle of it:

> [Frieda's] life was in evident danger, either from the risk of suicide or from exhaustion; somehow I had to break through. At last I told her how painful her distress was, not only to herself and to her family, but to me. I said that no one could be near her in that state without being deeply affected; I felt sorrow with her, and for her, in her loss.
>
> The effect of this was instantaneous, and very great.[24]

As Lacan points out in his seminar *Angoisse*, it is an indication of how far Little was pushed that in this way, she was able to take on, that is, assume responsibility for, love.[25] In other words, and to put it less intimately, she was able to assume responsibility for the transference. And what became evident at that point was not just Little's frustration but her anxiety, not Frieda's anxiety, her own. Pushed to the limit, without thinking about what she was doing, and dispensing with interpretation, Little "goes all out."[26]

Little's difficulties and her eventual response to them confirm Lacan's aphorism that resistance is always on the side of the analyst. It is the analyst who is resistant to taking up what Lacan refers to, in the seminar *Angoisse*, as "the place of lack in the analysis."[27] This place can also be understood as the place, in the analysis, of failure, the failure, that is, of the sexual relation.

Now, let me be clear here. In company with Lacan, I am not offering Little's case as a model of a psychoanalytic treatment. Most especially, I am not suggesting

23 Little, M. (1957). 'R'—The analyst's total response to his patient's needs. In: *The International Journal of Psychoanalysis*, vol. 38, no. 3–4, pp. 240–254.
24 Little, M. (1957). 'R'—The analyst's total response to his patient's needs, p. 247.
25 Lacan, J. (2014 [1963]). *Anxiety*, p. 143.
26 Little, M. (1957). 'R'—The analyst's total response to his patient's needs, p. 245.
27 Lacan, J. (2014 [1963]). *Anxiety*, p. 143.

that we abandon the psychoanalytic method and retreat to some sort of empathic, self-oriented psychotherapy.

Reading Little with Lacan, we can see that her interventions, that is, her exceptional interventions, as opposed to her many rather routine interpretations, are the opposite of such a retreat. Nor were these interventions prompted by empathy. They were prompted by anxiety, her own. And that anxiety was, in turn, prompted by the fact that, forgetting herself, including her self, as analyst, she found herself submitted to that anxiety at its highest point.

For Frieda, the sudden death of her friend Ilse constituted a lapse in the logic of the universe. For Lacan, the impossibility of the sexual relation can be understood as just such a lapse but by way of writing. As he puts in his seminar *Encore*, it is a lapse which only shows itself in the negative: It doesn't stop not being written.[28]

What turned the tables in Frieda's analysis was her analyst's courage. Putting herself aside, that is, the self, in the form of that carapace known as the analyst's suit of clothing, what Little demonstrated was a capacity to encounter this place of failure.

❦ ❦ ❦

Finally, I want to propose that this also turns the tables for Lacan and even as he was pushing through them towards Duras in that encounter around midnight in a murky subterranean bar in Paris. In the moment of that cry, "You don't know what you are saying," there is a lapse in the logic of the universe. Lacan, too, forgets himself.

What he is on the verge of encountering in that moment is not Duras but, once again, the impossible. This time, however, the impossible takes the form of She, The Woman, The Woman who does not stop, *not* being written, The Woman who, being Not-All-There, does not exist.

This is madness, the madness of the analyst.

28 Lacan, J. (1998 [1973]). *On Feminine Sexuality*, p. 94 (session of 20.3.73).

Part II

Disavowal . . . not without anxiety

Chapter 5

Lacan's Sadean reading of jouissance

Linda Clifton

> I had the skin of the cunt.[1]

> There are bloody corpses everywhere, infants torn from their mothers' arms, young women with their throats cut after an orgy, cups full of blood and wine, unimaginable tortures. Cauldrons are heated, racks set up, skulls broken, men flayed alive: there is shouting, swearing, blasphemy; hearts are ripped from bodies: all this on every line. What a scoundrel he is! In his first book [Justine] he shows us a poor girl at bay, lost, ruined, shrinking under a rain of blows, led by inhuman monsters through one underground vault after another, from graveyard to graveyard, beaten, broken, devoured alive, wilting, crushed [. . .] when the author has committed every crime there is, when he is sated with incest and monstrosities, when he stands panting above the corpses he has stabbed and violated, when there is no church he has not sullied, no child he has not sacrificed to his rage, no moral thought on which he has not flung the foulness of his own thoughts and words, then at last this man pauses, looks at himself, smiles to himself and is not frightened.[2]

These words of outrage published in 1834 are those of a French writer and critic, apparently now forgotten, Jules Janin. The author in question, who is not frightened in the face of his own exploits, is the Marquis de Sade.

In a kind of Sadean twist, Janin is incited in his outrage to flay his reader with the visceral horrors of the Sadean text. One can be flayed by words as one can be flayed by whips. For Janin, it seems there is little or no difference. Sade the author is Sade the criminal who "stands panting above the corpses he has stabbed and violated." The act of writing becomes an exploitative act. Sade the writer becomes Sade the murderer. Writing as an assault. Could we say writing as a penetrative act?

This passage is quoted by Georges Bataille in his *Eroticism to* exemplify the reaction to Sade's writings of the one designated by Bataille as the normal man, the

1 Cited in Lacan, J. (1962–1963). *The Seminar of Jacques Lacan Book X Anxiety*. C. Gallagher (Trans.). London: Karnac Books, session of 6.3.63.
2 Janin, J. cited in Bataille, G. (2012 [1957]). *Eroticism*. London: Penguin Modern Classics, p. 177.

DOI: 10.4324/9781003712480-7

man of reason, the "anxious man whose first reaction is to de Sade as his daughter's potential murderer."[3]

As outlined in a previous paper, Sade with Lacan, Sade's writing was lifted from the suppression of two centuries by Guillame Apollinaire, early in the twentieth century.[4] By the 1950s and '60s, it was being lionised by numerous French intellectuals—Bataille, Klossowski, Paulhan, de Beauvoir, Barthes, Foucault. It is in this context that Lacan writes what everyone agrees is a difficult text, Kant avec Sade.[5]

What is the value of Lacan's difficult text, and why should we submit ourselves to the even more difficult task of enduring a reading of Sade which, as Bataille points out, makes the normal man, the man of reason, anxious, in fear for his own daughter's life?

We can find a preliminary answer to these questions in David Pereira's proposal in 2012, in his Melbourne Seminar Psychoanalysis, Philosophy and Theology, that Lacan deepens his own explorations of jouissance by making a Sadean reading of jouissance. It is a reading which conveys an extensive and complex analysis of the Sadean project, neither celebrating Sadean atrocities nor espousing their supposed freedoms. In his Sadean reading of jouissance, Lacan highlights something touched on in Bataille's rendition of the normal man confronting Sade. Bataille's normal man reading Sade is suffused with anxiety. Lacan's reading of Sade highlights the proximity of jouissance and anxiety.

In this return to Lacan's reading of Sade, it is the proximity of jouissance and anxiety that will be highlighted, a proximity of relevance to the contemporary psychoanalytic clinic.

Lacan insists on the value of a Sadean reading. Why does he consider that we should not spare ourselves?

In his Seminar *The Ethics of Psychoanalysis* [1959–60], Lacan says the following about Sade's writing:

> It has been called an unsurpassable body of work, in the sense that it achieves an absolute of the unbearable in what can be expressed in words relative to the transgression of all human limits.
>
> [. . .] in no other literature, at no other time has there been such a scandalous body of work. No one else has done such injury to the feelings and thoughts of mankind.

Thus, as Maurice Blanchot puts it, "Isn't that a reason for us to be interested in it?"

> [O]ne cannot conceive of an atrocity that isn't to be found in Sade's catalogue. The assault on one's sensibility is of a kind to be literally stupefying: in other words one loses one's bearings.[6]

3 Bataille, G. (2012 [1957]). *Eroticism*, p. 179.

4 Clifton, L. (1992). Sade with Lacan. In: *Homage to Lacan: Papers of the Freudian School of Melbourne*. F. Bagot, L. Clifton and D. Pereira (Eds.). The Freudian School of Melbourne.

5 Lacan, J. [1963 (2006)]. Kant with Sade. In *Ecrits: The First Complete Edition in English*. B. Fink (Trans.). New York & London: W. W. Norton & Co.

6 Lacan, J. (1992 [1959–1960]). *The Seminar of Jacques Lacan Book VII: The Ethics of Psychoanalysis*. J.-A. Miller (Ed.), D. Porter (Trans.), pp. 200–201.

The reason that the book falls from one's hands is nothing else but "the response of a being, whether reader or writer, at the approach to a centre of incandescence or an absolute zero that is physically unbearable."[7]

Why is Lacan interested in this centre of incandescence or an absolute zero which is physically unbearable? Can we hear an answer in the way he describes jouissance as presenting itself "as buried at the centre of a field [with] the characteristics of inaccessibility, obscurity and opacity?" This field is

> surrounded by a barrier which makes access to it difficult for the subject to the point of inaccessibility, because jouissance appears not purely and simply as the satisfaction of a need but as satisfaction of a drive."[8]

As I read it, this is the field that Sade attempted to storm two centuries earlier. It was this field of jouissance that Sade wanted to colonise, proposing the elimination of all forms of restraint on human conduct and a universal right of enjoyment to men and women of each other's bodies. This Sadean right of enjoyment is the logical extension of one of the literal meanings of jouissance—the rights of an enjoyment over.

Let's hear how Lacan develops his jouissance.

In 1966 in a lecture to doctors and psychoanalysts entitled Psychoanalysis and Medicine, Lacan said:

> What I call jouissance—in the sense in which the body experiences itself—is always in the nature of tension, in the sense of a forcing, of a spending, even of an exploit. Unquestionably there is jouissance at the level at which pain begins to appear and we know that it is only at this level of pain that a whole dimension of the organism which would otherwise remain veiled, can be experienced.[9]

In 1971 in Seminar 18 *On a Discourse That Might Not Be a Semblance,* he wrote:

> [T]he stuff of every enjoyment is close to suffering, this is even how we recognise how it is dressed up. If the plant was not manifestly suffering we would not know it was alive."[10]

7 Lacan, J. (1992 [1959–1960]). *The Seminar of Jacques Lacan Book VII*, p. 201.

8 Lacan, J. (1992 [1959–1960]). *The Seminar of Jacques Lacan Book VII*, p. 209.

9 Lacan, J. (1966 [2003]). Cited in Braunstein, N. (2003). Desire and jouissance in the teachings of Lacan. In *The Cambridge Companion to Lacan*. J.-M. Rabate (Ed.). London: Cambridge University Press, p. 103.

10 Lacan, J. (1971). *The Seminar of Jacques Lacan Book XVIII On a Discourse That Might Not Be a Semblance*. C. Gallagher (Trans.). London: Karnac Books, session of 17.3.71.

In 1972 in *Seminar XX Encore*:

> Isn't that precisely what psychoanalytic experience presupposes? The substance of the body on the condition that I defined it only as that which enjoys itself (*se jouit*) [. . .]
>
> [. . .] we don't know what it is to be alive except for the following fact, that a body is something that enjoys itself (*cela se jouit*).
>
> It enjoys itself by "corporizing" (*corporiser*) the body in a signifying way.
>
> [. . .] As is emphasised admirably by the kind of Kantian that Sade was, one can only enjoy a part of the Other's body, for the simple reason that one has never seen a body completely wrap itself around the Other's body to the point of surrounding it and phagocytizing it. That is why we must confine ourselves to simply giving it a little squeeze, like that, taking a forearm or anything else—ouch!
>
> Enjoying (*jouir*) has the property that it is, ultimately, one person's body that enjoys a part of the Other's body. But that part also enjoys—the Other likes it more or less, but it is a fact that the Other cannot remain indifferent to it.
>
> Occasionally something even happens [. . .] that is marked by utter signifying ambiguity—for the expression "enjoyment of the body" (*jouir du corps*) includes a genitive that has a certain Sadean flavor to it [. . .] or, on the contrary, an ecstatic, subjective flavor suggesting [. . .] that it is the Other who enjoys.[11]

The little demonstration that Lacan makes in front of his seminar audience, his squeezing of his arm and his "ouch!" shows the Sadean slide into cruelty that can occur when bodies begin to touch bodies. Here, the concept of jouissance is anchored in the body, in the body experiencing pain. In this and through the underlining of a tension, a forcing, an exploit, we are not far from Sade.

We arrive to Sadean cruelty and suffering in the following account of a passage in Sade highlighted by Lacan in Seminar X Anxiety in the seminar of March 6, 1963 where

> the characters, completely occupied in slaking on their chosen victims their greed for torments, enter into this bizarre, singular and curious trance [. . .] which is expressed in these strange words [. . .] "I had," cries the tormentor, "I had the skin of the cunt."

In Lacan's dazzling analysis of this passage he proposes that

> something is sought which is in a way the reverse of the subject, which takes on here its signification from this feature of the glove turned inside out which

11 Lacan, J. (1998 [1972–1973]). *Encore: The Seminar of Jacques Lacan Book XX*. J.-A. Miller (Ed.), B. Fink (Trans.). W.W. Norton & Company, pp. 23–24.

> underlines the feminine essence of the victim. It is the passage to what is outside of what is most hidden that is involved: but let us observe at the same time that this moment is in a way indicated in the text as being totally unpenetrated by the subject, allowing there precisely to be masked [. . .] the trait of his own anxiety.
>
> The sadist, the tormentor, the torturer, the agent is reduced to an instrument.
>
> That which in a way is hidden, except in a flash [. . .] the aim of his action is the work aspect of his operation. He also has a relationship with God [. . .] He cannot take a step forward without this reference to the supremely wicked being [. . .]
>
> . . . he goes to all sorts of exhausting trouble [. . .] to realise the jouissance of God.[12]

What Lacan conveys here in his reading of this bizarre scene is the tormentor's complete unknowing of what he seeks, of what drives him to the action he has taken or the words he utters. The skin of the cunt is offered as a moment of triumph, a making visible that which is hidden, a sacrifice of the woman in her feminine essence, to use Lacan's words, to the jouissance of the Other. The victim, always a woman for Sade, is penetrated and God knows what else. But the tormentor remains unpenetrated, masking his own anxiety.

This most extreme and bizarre sexual act was the product, as far as we know, of Sade's imagination, not his actual sexual practice. Strangely, it has a relevance to the contemporary psychoanalytic clinic through the analysis made of it by Lacan.

Of course, much is spoken in the contemporary clinic of bodies and sexualities, of orifices—their excitement and their pain—of penetrating and being penetrated, of orgasms and the absence of orgasms, of potency and its failures, of sexual ease and sexual disease, even of Sadean experimentation. But the relevance of Sade to the contemporary clinic is not in the Sadean or other practices that might be spoken of but in Lacan's analysis, where he proposes a proximity of jouissance and anxiety and its relation to penetration.

Lacan's analysis of this most extreme penetrative act allows me to propose the importance of this proximity of jouissance and anxiety to the contemporary clinic. The Sadean tormentor, while penetrating his victim, remains unpenetrated. His anxiety remains masked. In the abstinence of the psychoanalytic clinic, as in writing, it is only the word that can penetrate. What I take from Lacan via Sade is that to be penetrated, but really, not necessarily literally, is to allow an unmasking of anxiety. Not the moment of triumph of the Sadean tormentor, whose anxiety remains masked, but a moment of unmasking, of angst, difficult to bear for both analysand and analyst.

12 Lacan, J. (1962–1963). *The Seminar of Jacques Lacan Book X Anxiety*. C. Gallagher (Trans.). London: Karnac Books, session of 6.3.63.

Chapter 6

Me too

I know nothing

Megan Williams

My aim in this chapter is to examine two questions. The first is the complicity with which perverse acts are often greeted in society, in the form of widespread blindness to or silence about the perversion. The second is the relation of hysteria to perversion.

I am speaking of hysteria as a discourse—one which all of us speak at one time or another, notably in psychoanalysis. I wish to put forward that its relation to perversion unfolds in two moments. The second, more familiar moment is a denunciation of the perversion. It follows a first moment, of apparent consent to it. I say "apparent" because the speaker of the hysteric's discourse is divided—whether we take that to evoke Freud's well-known figure of the hysteric ripping her dress off with one hand whilst closing it over her with the other or remember that a subject may comply without knowing what it is that is being consented to. "Consent" in the Discourse of Hysteria, as defined by Lacan, concerns the hysteric's unconscious desire to produce knowledge about sexuality by following one who seems to know.[1]

Freud used the term "perversion" in two ways, as Maria-Ines Zentner also observes.[2] He first regarded it as definitive of subjectivity as such (the "polymorphous perversion" of infantile sexuality) and later as a psychopathological structure.[3,4] Arguments have been made for and against regarding perversion as a subjective structure in psychoanalytic terms. I do not enter here into that debate but rather speak from the position that an act may be taken as perverse if it falls within Lacan's characterisation of a pervert's act as one which produces subjective division—castration, in other words—in the partner.[5] That is, as Clavreul observes,

1 Lacan, J. (2007). *The Seminar of Jacques Lacan, Book XVII: The Other Side of Psychoanalysis*. R. Grigg (Trans.). New York & London: W. W. Norton & Co.

2 Zentner, M.-I. (1981). A Pseudonym, the itinerary for a perversion. In: *Papers of the Freudian School of Melbourne: Homage to Freud/On Perversion 1980*, p. 66.

3 Freud, S. (1905). Three essays on the theory of sexuality. SE VII.

4 Freud, S. (1939a [1940]). Splitting of the ego in the process of defence. SE XXIII.

5 Lacan, J. (1962–1963). *The Seminar of Jacques Lacan, Book X, Anxiety*. C. Gallagher (Trans.). Unpublished manuscript, session of 6.3.63.

DOI: 10.4324/9781003712480-8

anxiety and jouissance are forced into the space of the subject, but the subject is the partner, not the one who acts, the latter being rather in the position of instrument or object.[6] The perverse act forces the partner to experience anxiety and jouissance beyond what they can know or tolerate, so that it divides them and, in doing so, disavows castration on the side of the actor.

Complicity

Once upon a time, a lecturer in psychology at a well-known university was renowned for giving what came to be called "sex lectures," where he spoke about sex in everyday terms and in graphic detail, showed explicit photos, demonstrated his own tactile preferences by tracing them on a dick pic, and on one occasion reportedly showed a 20-minute video of sexual intercourse between the members of a couple he was treating for sexual problems. He had affairs with some students which "everyone" knew about, and others he either propositioned or engaged with in ways that would nowadays be called "grooming." His essential trait was that *he knew*—he knew with certainty how to produce or correct sexual enjoyment, in the clinic and elsewhere, and he disseminated this knowledge in self-help books and in therapy sessions, where he instructed student therapists exactly what to say to their clients through earbuds from the other side of a one-way window.

Curiously, no-one seems to have denounced this behaviour as perverse at the time, at least not publicly, and not for many years, years during which the psychologist left that university and went on to write more self-help books, begin a private practice, give clinical advice on radio and television, function as resident psychologist of a reality TV show, and become president of the Australian Psychological Society. He consulted to the Department of Human Services on the risk to society of paedophiles seeking parole, where reputedly, his reports typically concluded that the risk of re-offending was low (contradicting statistical evidence). He also founded and directed a new university psychology department—employed to do this by another psychologist who was later convicted of paedophilia.

Many years later, he was himself convicted and jailed for having, as a young psychologist and scout leader forty years previously, groomed, molested, and raped a number of young boys. The reporting of this in the press was rather muted—his disgrace did not achieve the magnitude of his fame.

I was brought to this chapter by listening to the ABC radio program, *Background Briefing*, on this psychologist's eventual conviction, very late in his life, for historic child sexual abuse. Hearing the interviews which testified to his notoriety as a young lecturer at his first university and the concerns which people now claimed to have had at the time, I wondered about the silence back then of all of us who witnessed his parading of a sexual knowledge that others didn't

6 Clavreul, J. (1980). The perverse couple. In: *Returning to Freud: Clinical Psychoanalysis in the School of Lacan*. S. Schneiderman (Ed.). CT: Yale University Press, pp. 220–221.

have. I suspect that this promise of knowledge is what seduced us. He had been much talked about, either as a curiosity or as a knowledgeable expert, a liberal, a radical free of neurotic repressions. Observers had thus worked to account for his behaviour in the terms of the Master Discourse, aided by the fact that it was difficult to determine by what standard his acts could be judged as wrong. Freud, in his final paper on perversion, alludes to a similar difficulty when he finds himself uncertain as to whether he is reporting something long familiar or new and puzzling, and Octave Mannoni consciously echoes this remark in saying of perversion: "one finds oneself torn between an impression of extreme banality and a powerful feeling of strangeness."[7,8] What we heard from the psychologist's famous "sex lectures" had frequently seemed to be no more than a banal observation or piece of advice amounting to common sense, yet his claim to command desire as if it were caused by a possessed or obtainable object, owing nothing to lack, amounts to a disavowal of a castration—a castration which is nevertheless evoked by the very multiplicity of his conquests. His presentation of himself as undivided, master of an absolute knowledge that owed nothing to the unconscious, was, psychoanalysis would tell us, an *imposture*, which functioned by his reduction of sexual knowledge to technical *know-how*. His listeners were largely unable to profit from his advice because, being divided, they enjoyed via their unconscious, but what was hidden—perhaps also from himself—is that he *knew how* to read their unconscious, and so could *make* them enjoy by the graphic displays which forced both jouissance and anxiety into the space of the watching subjects, a fact borne out by some of their testimonies.

Perhaps the most compelling reason why none of the watching audience spoke up publicly is articulated by Jean Clavreul when he comments that the essential of the perverse practice

> is that it retain enough verisimilitude to cause anguish and enough lack of verisimilitude and fantasy for it all to be interpreted as a play to which you can't take offence without appearing to be ridiculous.[9]

Apparently none of us was willing to take the risk of appearing ridiculous or prudish and reactionary, and so we lent ourselves to the circuit of perversion. Or was it more than that? It seems to me now that we who were our psychologist's silent audience said to ourselves the very thing that Freud has the pervert saying, characterised by Mannoni as: "Yes, I know well, but all the same . . ."—we said, "Yes, I know, what he does is over the top/embarrassing/egregious, but still, he seems to

7 Freud, S. (1939a [1940]). Splitting of the ego in the process of defence, p. 275.
8 Mannoni, O. (2003). *I Know Well, But All the Same . . . Perversion and the Social Relation. sic IV*, p. 70.
9 Clavreul, J. (1980). The perverse couple, p. 228.

know"—as if he had the secret to the sexual relation and could share it with us.[10] Clavreul is amongst others in observing that the pervert requires the presence of a third party, an Other who is there only in order to be disavowed: to be taken, in his blindness, as complicit or else exposed as impotent in representing the Law.[11] In our case, then, it may be that we students and staff collectively represented *the Other who is fascinated and thus debauched*—the impotent representative of the Law. This Other is essential to a perverse act defined in terms of a disavowal of castration—castration must not only be disavowed but be seen to be so; the actor be seen to have triumphed over the Law of subjectivity.

In the same context, we could evoke the recent events of our own Australian parliament: a young woman allegedly raped in the blind office of a cabinet minister; another minister who represents the law accused of historical rape and both the parliament and the law impotent to deal with the situation; multiple women subjected to sexual molestation, innuendo, and prejudice, which the institution is impotent to act on except by instituting "enquiries" which will produce knowledge that is structurally incapable, from the outset, of functioning as truth. Can we then say of contemporary discourse that the third party to its perversion is no longer the pervert's classical Other of priest, judge, or governor (representatives of one kind of law or another), but . . . us, the mass, the blind chorus that witnesses without knowing what we are seeing, in concert with the impotent bureaucracy of our institutions?

The question would seem to move the perverse act from the fringes of sexual encounter to a central position in our institutions. Here, referring back to Freud, we move to perversion taken not as individual psychopathology but as the structure of phallic sexuality—remembering that all subjects are inscribed here, not only males. Freud designated this as the polymorphous perversion of infantile sexuality and Lacan as the subject's relation with an object *a*, whose place will be taken by substitutes from infancy onwards, comprising *père-version* or the version/perversion of the father.[12] It follows the signification of the phallus given by the castration that is passed on from father to son.

From this perspective of *père-version* as characterising masculine sexuality, here is another story: Once upon a time, a young female senator arrives at a cabinet meeting whose present participants are all men and sits next to a male colleague she is friendly with. Calm and smiling, he reaches over, places his hand on her knee, and runs it up her thigh, then walks off. She freezes. At least some of the men present see this but say nothing, and neither does she. There is a multitude of similar accounts in the testimonies of female parliamentarians interviewed by journalist Annabelle Crabb for the Australian Broadcasting Commission documentary, *Ms*

10 Mannoni, O. (2003). *I Know Well, But All the Same*.

11 Mannoni, O. (2003). *I Know Well, But All the Same*, pp. 218–219.

12 Lacan, J. (1974–1975). *The Seminar of Jacques Lacan Book XXII R. S. I.* J. Stone (Trans.). Unpublished manuscript, session of 21.1.75.

Represented—of encountering misogyny, prejudice, or explicitly sexual comments and acts from their male counterparts and of remaining silent. The reasons given for the silence range from being transfixed by shock to the idea that in speaking, they would portray themselves as hysterical women to assuming that the attacks would pass once the novelty of having women parliamentarians wore off. These women had their own version of "yes, I know, but all the same"—"Yes, I know it's wrong and it makes me furious, but still, it's better for all women if I shut up and get on with the work and prove that I'm here on merit."

The Me Too movement testifies to thousands of women to whom these things happened and who remained silent. Who remained silent until, suddenly, they didn't: The silence of the first moment turns to the denunciation of the second. Prime Minister Gillard and Senator Hanson-Young famously and hysterically denounce their attackers in parliament—"hysterically" in that it falls structurally to the Discourse of Hysteria to denounce perversion. Brittany Higgins denounces a rape, and women everywhere say: "Me too." Many of the women interviewed by Annabelle Crabb recant their silence and say: *We were wrong; we should have spoken out.*

As Clavreul observes, once this pendulum has swung, the third party, too, opens its eyes and is horrified, scandalised, revolted—no longer able to act the voyeur once the secret is out.[13] Suddenly, there are public support, calls for action, and gestures of solidarity, much like the AFL world's about-face on racism after the sustained, public crushing of Indigenous player Adam Goodes. Politicians denounce as "disgusting" the acts that have been perpetrated over many years during which the same politicians apparently saw nothing amiss. The mass, the observing third party, apparently now disavows the memory of its silence, its seduction, its *Me too, I know nothing, see nothing.*

In sum, then, there can come a moment when the universal, structural *père-version* of masculine sexuality swings into acts which are properly perverse, as defined earlier. For this, the third party is necessary, the blind observer of the perversion of the law who, in seeing nothing amiss, gives his seal to the efficacity of the disavowing act. Even where there is no audience, the clinic suggests that the complicit third party is nevertheless there in fantasy.

Hysteria: from partner to denouncer

The second of my two questions concerns not the third party but the second, the partner to the perverse act—albeit a "partner" who may be more acted-upon than acting; who may be an unwitting victim. Why is it that hysteria first lends itself to perversion, only in a second moment to call it out? The question concerns the relation of the Discourse of Hysteria to knowledge or, more particularly, to truth, and to the disjunction between knowledge and truth. Perhaps it would not be inaccurate

13 Clavreul, J. (1980). The perverse couple, p. 219.

to say that the hysteric seeks truth via the one who appears as master of knowledge, only to be disappointed or worse.

A woman's subjectivity tends more towards hysteria than a male subject's because, insofar as the phallus represents her sexuality, it signifies her as an object. How is she to take up the place of an object—by assuming a semblance of the phallic object desired by masculine *père-version*—and where then is her own sexuality located? *Her own sexuality is located in the gap in the psyche*, the place empty of representations. This term comes from Freud's early account of the first encounter of a child with sexuality, where he observed that an obsessional subject, more usually male, is able to assume the experience of jouissance as his own. Even though it goes beyond pleasure into guilt, it affirms his narcissism via the father-perversion (*père-version*) which he inherits.[14] The hysteric, on the other hand, cannot represent this jouissance under the signification which the phallus gives her, so there remains a "gap in the psyche"—something experienced without being known, with the result that the truth of her sexuality can thereafter only be spoken as fiction.

Freud tells the story of a young woman, Emma, who spoke such a fiction, produced by the unconscious to fill the gap in the psyche created when she was molested through her clothes by a grinning man in a shop.[15] Using these signifiers, her unconscious explains her subsequent phobia by a story of boys in a shop having laughed at her clothes. We can all give accounts of girls who go with dangerous men or revisit sexual molesters and who never tell until their analyses, when often, they ask—without finding an answer—why they didn't tell. (I leave aside the silent third party of perversion: the mothers, fathers, and communities who saw nothing or who knew but disavowed their knowledge.) Like Emma, the hysteric gives many reasons for her silence or her return to the pervert, but we can hear these as dissimulations or fictions—the false premise or *proton pseudos* masking the gap in the psyche that Freud considered to characterise the hysteric's first encounter with sexuality.

Unable to assume this un-represented sexuality as *her* enjoyment, she might misrepresent it as something done *to* her by an other who is therefore accused of perversion. To say that this is a mis(Ms)-representation is not to say that it is factually untrue—indeed, it usually corresponds to the facts—but rather to say that it fails to adequately represent the truth of her own sexuality, the truth she perhaps sought in acceding to the perverse partner. If it answers the adequation requirement of truth, it nevertheless fails as aletheia, disclosure. If she seeks knowledge of this truth from a master of knowledge, what is produced is unable to be thought and yet is experienced: a gap in *her* psyche. And thus, unlike the paranoiac, she cannot entirely disown the experience: It forms part of her psyche, even as an unknown;

14 Freud, S. (1892). Draft K the neuroses of defence (A Christmas Fairy Tale). In: *Extracts from the Flies Papers*. SE I: 220–229.

15 Freud, S. (1950 [1895]). Project for a scientific psychology. SE 1: 353–355.

even if not part of her *me*. Her seeking knowledge has divided her again, which is exactly what the perverse act seeks to do.

Hopefully, it will be clear from the foregoing that by "hysteria" I am not evoking the casual, popular dismissal of claims of sexual abuse as "hysterical," meaning untrue—though that usage is in itself pertinent in demonstrating how integrally hysteria is linked to the notion of truth and in evoking the way in which, historically, hysterics have spoken *truth without knowledge*: without knowing what they are saying, as Emma first spoke the *truth* of her molestation with a phobic symptom and a fictional story.

Let's consider with Lacan, then, that in the *Discourse* of Hysteria, a speaker troubled by this division asks a supposed master of knowledge about it. The master offers her masses of knowledge, but it's not what she wants to know, which is *the truth* of the sexual relation. Constrained by his own discourse, the master can only act towards her according to her signified place in it (as object), which is what the cabinet minister did so crudely with the woman senator. It is the pervert who can penetrate her with truth, but not a truth that can be assumed as knowledge, since what he commands is the traumatic truth of a jouissance which, along with anxiety, only recreates a gap in her psyche. This is not what she has consented to, and she may even come to denounce it. Nevertheless, her search for knowledge may have first led her to consent to the apparent promise of knowledge contained in his offer.

If this promise makes the pervert a natural—that is, discursive—partner for the hysteric, the obverse is not the case. The pervert is attracted to those who, in Clavreul's terms, "incarnate a value venerated socially."[16] Yet there is one figure of the hysteric's discourse who does incarnate such a value: the virgin, innocent of sexual knowledge, divided between the value that desire takes in its familial route and the unconscious erotism that inhabits the gap in her consciousness, an erotism which Freud observes was once taboo.

Does initiation into that sexuality require a moment of perversion? Freud's "neurotica" held this to be the case until he flinched at the consequence that all fathers would then have to be regarded as perverse.[17] The "Taboo of Virginity" tells us that the initiation of a virgin into sexuality used to be assigned to someone outside the social structures that the girl belongs to, who will brave the danger that is to be awakened in order to take the erotic outside the socius and the subject, so that the girl may safely enter the phallic circuit of Eros, marriage, and children, the paternal made safe, locking away the gap in the psyche, leaving the encounter between the erotic girl and the perverse father relegated to fantasy.[18]

16 Clavreul, J. (1980). The perverse couple, p. 220.

17 Freud, S. (1897). Letter 69. In: *Extracts from the Fliess Papers*. SE I: 259–260.

18 Freud, S. (1918). The taboo of virginity (Contributions to the Psychology of Love III). SE XI: 191–208.

Smooth Talk

This year, the Melbourne International Film Festival screened a film from 1985 entitled *Smooth Talk*, in which a young Laura Dern plays adolescent virgin Connie, luminescent with a sexuality that she is only partly aware of yet is driven to awaken, impatient with the domesticity of her family and her childish place in it, at odds with her mother and compliant older sister, and dismissive of her boyish father.[19] Her family cannot initiate her into sexuality: We see her father make his gaze blind and retreat from her sexuality when he misrepresents the danger of her entering a bar full of men in a miniskirt (which he happened to observe) as that of crossing the highway in traffic. Her mother, having failed to restore the cuddly, childish Connie, displays her envy, her unsatisfied sexuality, and her disappointment with her assigned place in the phallic circuit by dancing all alone to Connie's music. And Connie's older sister, June, complicit with the father's impotence, has become a good, sensible, apparently asexual adult: She has entered the phallic circuit and locked away the gap in the psyche.

Lying to her mother, Connie goes with her girlfriend to the mall to experiment with how to attract boys. In front of her bedroom mirror, she tries out revealing clothes and looks and flirty talk. That is, we see her calling on a gaze that will sexualise her in this way that is foreign to her, divided between a shy awkwardness and an erotism given into the other's keeping. One night, she and her friend dare to brave the burger bar across the divide of the highway, where the older boys and girls hang out and make out. Echoing Freud's classical figure of hysteria, she wears her sexy top but, taking fright at what it reveals of something she doesn't know in herself, she covers it with a baggy jacket, which her friend nevertheless pulls off her as they enter. She sits at the bar, awkward, squirming, skinny and angular, her face grimacing as though in pain. Yet something in her knows how to seduce. Over a few nights, a routine develops where a boy approaches her, they talk, she gets into his car, and they drive somewhere and make out. She always leaves before it goes too far. Trying to speak of what she is discovering to her sister, she says, "It feels so good when they hug me, so soft." But this is Eros: being loved, finding a phallic reflection of herself in being desired, withdrawing before she becomes an object of jouissance. This is Dora. It isn't initiation. Initiation is when it *does* go too far, beyond what she has known or desired, to the trauma of the cause: the truth that lacks representation. For that, she requires a perverse act.

Arnold is the smooth talker of the title, a man rather than a boy, who sees Connie on that first night and marks her with a pointing finger as his. He doesn't pursue her immediately but takes his time, watching her, finding out all about her and her family, and then making his move. One afternoon, when he knows that she will be

19 *Smooth Talk*. (1985). J. Copra (Dir.), T. Cole (screenplay). Adapted from short story Oates, J. C. (1966). *Where Are You Going, Where Have You Been?* Distribution: Goldcrest Films, International Spectrafilm.

at home alone, he drives to her house, accompanied by a silent friend who stays in the car plugged into his transistor, representing the suborned big Other, the complicit third party. When Connie opens the door to Arnold, he speaks with immediate familiarity, from which she backs away in fright and astonishment, saying, "But I don't know you!" telling him to leave, that her family will be back, yet not able to close the door in his face. Already hooked by his knowing, her face twists and distorts in an effort to grasp his discourse, to articulate what it is that's wrong with it, since ostensibly, he is only visiting, respectfully waiting outside the door. He takes advantage of every hesitancy, moving smoothly from familiarity to the appearance of intimacy: "You're my lover. You will be. I know. I know lots of things—I know all about you." Clavreul observes, "the perverse structure permits him to glow in such a way that the person listening always feels more or less threatened," and Connie responds to his menace by telling him that she will call the police, but she can't bring herself to do so, since he hasn't done anything wrong.[20] And he goes on talking in a calm and friendly voice, acknowledging her fright as an obstacle they both face rather than as caused by him, speaking as an older friend and advisor, which increases her anxiety and bewilderment. At one point, she sits just out of his sight in the hallway, holding the phone in her lap, crying and whispering, "Mum" but still not phoning anyone. Patient and knowing, Arnold speaks as though he and she both *know* what is already written:

> You're scared. It's natural. You're going to come out that door and come for a ride with me. This is going to happen, Connie, you and I both know it, and you're going to be brave and I'm going to help you. Come on out now—it's better that you come out on your own. I don't want to come in there into your home where I don't belong.

And she does! Here is the moment when something unconscious in her takes him for a master of knowledge. She stands up and walks out of the door and follows him to his car, where he courteously opens the door for her and they drive off. She is "impotent to be anything other than consenting" because he reads her unconscious and knows "which signifiers imprison [her, which she] cannot extricate [herself] from. He will use this knowledge to make [her] attain summits of anxiety and jouissance."[21]

We don't see what happens—the gap in the psyche is maintained—but we see them arrive back some time later. She has crossed a threshold, has been initiated by the outsider who dared the taboo of virginity, and she has no further use of him nor he of her. He leans across her to push open her door and silently waits for her to get out. As she walks past him she says, "Don't you ever come back around here again." He smiles, shrugs.

20 Clavreul, J. (1980). The perverse couple, p. 232.
21 Clavreul, J. (1980). The perverse couple, p. 221.

Later, she tries to assimilate the gap in the psyche into the social-familial, phallic discourse by speaking to her sister, but June reacts to the first words—"I went with a boy"—with such horror that she shuts up, shuts the door, dissimulates, says she was joking. *It never happened.* She will not speak of it again. The potential moment for building a fictional representation, a proton pseudos, has passed.

She may still reach a moment of conclusion and act. Perhaps, a long way down the track, Arnold will get himself arrested for rape, and the whole, blind town, the complicit Other, will suddenly be righteously up in arms, and Connie will join the girls who come forward to say, "Me too." It will give her legitimacy of a kind as a victim—will mask the gap in the psyche with a kind of identity—but it will not be a knowledge capable of rejoining her truth.

Conclusion

Implicit here is the notion that a female subject is always initially virgin in relation to what inhabits the gap in her psyche, even though that gap was created by something first experienced. Am I proposing that it takes a perverse act to awaken it, to initiate her into a sexuality in which she might take it as her own? I am saying that it is one way, perhaps even the most common way, because the irruption of jouissance into the space of the subject of speech and language is always traumatic. That which has remained a gap in the psyche is Other to her—as we see so clearly when Connie calls on the gazes of the mirror and the burger bar boys to sexualise her or when she follows Arnold to his car, possessed by the perverse logic of his words. The Discourse of Hysteria concerns this thing which remains Other, as does the taboo of virginity, though each does so in opposite ways. The taboo operates on the side of the Discourse of the Master, the phallic discourse, which assigns no place to feminine sexuality—the phallus being All—and in which a woman can only be located as object.[22] Hence the "primitive" practices referred to by Freud, which call on the outsider to take aside the erotic excess, leaving the female subject to the roles of wife and mother—this is not an initiation into her own sexuality but an induction into the phallic order. Of a similar order are the perverse practices that relegate femininity to a place as object (the rape in parliament, the senator who ran his hand up the leg of his colleague) or exclude it as dangerous, excessive, or uncanny (a male parliamentarian who sniffed the seat of a female colleague after she stood up; Senator David Leyonhjelm telling Senator Sarah Hanson-Young to "stop shagging men"; Prime Minister Julia Gillard referred to as a witch, barren of womb and pantry). The Discourse of Hysteria, on the other hand, denounces

22 This point is made in differing ways in Lacan, J. (2002 [1958]). The signification of the phallus. In: *Écrits: The First Complete Edition in English*. B. Fink (Trans.). New York & London: W. W. Norton & Co., and later in Lacan, J. (1999 [1972–1973]). *On Feminine Sexuality, the Limits of Love and Knowledge: Encore, the Seminar of Jacques Lacan Book XX*. J.-A. Miller (Ed.), B. Fink (Trans.). New York & London: W. W. Norton & Co., chapters VI, VII.

this disavowal of feminine sexuality. Nevertheless, it addresses itself to the wrong place, to the master supposed to know, the phallic other, and then rejects the answer that it receives, since the master discourse, whether perverse or not, can only signify her as object. That is, hysteria begins by going to an other's place in order to find out something about itself—which is what Freud observed when he said that the hysteric identifies with a man in order to find out about desire, or Lacan, when he said that hysteria makes the man. These ways of calling on the phallic discourse to provide knowledge tend towards closing the gap in the psyche, whether they aim to do so or not.

Perversion can open it—many testimonies confirm this in their use of words like "shock" and "trauma"—these words refer to jouissance. So too can the discourse of the psychoanalyst—and its closeness to perversion has been noted before. Only in psychoanalysis, the hysteric asks the question of an other supposed-to-know who *does not answer* the question but *returns it to the Other within herself*, which may potentially penetrate the gap in the psyche. This is an awakening for which she herself is response-able: which only she can find her own way of taking up. This opens the possibility of doing something other than sealing the gap with a fiction or with the identity of a victim.

Part III

In praise of hysteria—Symposium in honour of Moustapha Safouan

Chapter 7

Introducing the work of Moustapha Safouan

A writing of letters—de lettres

Tine Nørregaard

In 1981, four years after the foundation of the Freudian School of Melbourne, we find in the third volume of the *Papers of the Freudian School of Melbourne* an introduction by Oscar Zentner to two seminars held in the School by Moustapha Safouan at the time, one entitled On Symbolism, the other On Jokes:

> The only way the Freudian School has of presenting Dr. Safouan is to make quite clear something we said at our last Homage to Freud in September, when we knew that Dr. Lacan had died. We said at the time that when a real analyst dies the School does not make a single minute of silence. The School produces a work and today's seminar is really this confirmation.[1]

Today, it is Moustapha Safouan we pay homage to, a real analyst who has died, and the Symposium is a response to this loss: We don't stay silent, but we work; a work produced from transference.

Moustapha Safouan was an analyst born in Egypt who took part in Lacan's first seminars in 1953, and he continued to work with Lacan until the end. He was a training analyst with the Société française de psychanalyse in Strasbourg until the split that led Lacan to found L'École freudienne de Paris in 1964. Safouan also bore witness to the experience of being present in the time of Lacan's invention of the procedure of the pass; he was an Analyst of the School (Analyste de L'École) in L'École freudienne de Paris until its dissolution in 1980, as well as being part of the Jury of the Pass during this time. Safouan has visited the Freudian School of Melbourne twice, and several of his papers have been printed in the *Papers of the Freudian School of Melbourne*. The work of Safouan thus forms part of the psychoanalytic discourse which has been produced in the School since its inception, and his seminars and papers give witness to his particular transference to Lacan as well as to his participation in a time in history that has shaped the Lacanian

1 Safouan, M. (1982). Seminar I—On symbolism. In: *Papers of the Freudian School of Melbourne: Homage to Freud: On Angst*. O. Zentner (Ed.). Melbourne: The Freudian School of Melbourne, p. 83.

DOI: 10.4324/9781003712480-10

discourse of psychoanalysis. It offers an address to an important otherness beyond the School in the transferences which pertain to the ongoing writing of the psychoanalytic discourse.

To be bitten by words and allow himself to be perturbed by the effects of different languages seems indeed central to Safouan's own transference to psychoanalysis. He grew up in Alexandria during the period leading up to the Second World War, a period he regarded as the "epoch of letters," rich with the influence of great Arabic poets at the time, which for Safouan was like being "drowned in letters."[2] He left Egypt to study philosophy at the Sorbonne in Paris, where he undertook an analysis that became didactic while he also took part in Lacan's early seminars. As he mentioned in an interview in 2012, "I liked psychoanalysis and the way I experienced discoveries of how I was a victim of words."[3] Safouan notes that Lacan never tried to teach him anything, and he describes his transference to Lacan with the Arabic word *Al-Mourid* [the desiring one].[4] For Safouan, this desire is a gift that is driven by a continuous want to know that is never satisfied.

Safouan translated Freud's *The Interpretation of Dreams* into classical Arabic in 1953 during a period of time in which he was forced to stay in Egypt due to Nasser's coup d'état. He notes that this was a work that immersed him in language to find a way to translate the style of Freud's writing into the style spoken amongst the sheiks and professors in the culture of the cafés in Cairo at the time.[5] This impact of the translation of the unconscious Safouan considers is central to the desire of the analyst.[6] There is then a question which arises at the end of the analysis: Why does one want to repeat this experience of a translation of the unconscious with the unconscious of someone else?[7] This is the same question as the one which asks what has made this particular analysis didactic.

Throughout his work, Safouan continued to consider the structure of the Oedipus complex in relation to the law and jouissance as the point of transmission of the father. Since the paternal position in the structure of the family is different today than at the beginning of psychoanalysis, Safouan proposes that "we are at the end of psychoanalysis since we are at the end of the Oedipus complex."[8] Such a rather provoking proposition demands each analyst to continue to question psychoanalysis

2 MacCabe, C. (2012). Interview with Moustapha Safouan. In: *Zamyn: Anthropology of Corporations*. https://www.zamyn.org/interviews/maccabe-safouan/interview.html.

3 MacCabe, C. (2012). Interview with Moustapha Safouan.

4 Plon, M. and Samovault, T. (2017). Grand entretien avec Moustapha Safouan, 9 mai, 2017. In: *En attendant Nadeau, Journal de la littérature, des idées et des arts. Numéro 32*. https://www.en-attendant-nadeau.fr/2017/05/09/grand-entretien-safouan/. [My trans.].

5 MacCabe, C. (2012). Interview with Moustapha Safouan.

6 Safouan, M. (1994). Jacques Lacan and the question of the training of analysts. In: *Papers of the Freudian School of Melbourne. Lacanian Psychoanalytic Writings: The Lacanian School*, vol. 15, D. Pereira (Ed.), C. Schneider (Trans.). Melbourne: The Freudian School of Melbourne, pp. 133–134.

7 Safouan, M. (1994). Jacques Lacan and the question of the training of analysts.

8 Plon, M. and Samovault, T. (2017). Grand entretien avec Moustapha Safouan, 9 mai, 2017. [My translation].

and their function from the field of the symbolic and language in which the discourse of psychoanalysis is produced. It is in essence a question of how the law is tied with symbolic castration and the function of the father in the contingencies of the life of each subject. It is from the imprint of the contingencies of his own life, the one he was born into, and the one he chose to live in as an analyst who allowed himself to be immersed in several cultures and languages, that Safouan considers the Oedipus complex as just one of many cultural forms which effect symbolic castration in the subject.[9]

The title of this Symposium In Praise of Hysteria is also the title of a paper of Safouan's from 1974 in which he raises a question about how we may understand the relationship between the law and the function of the father in the structure of hysteria today.[10] Safouan's praise is a return to Freud through Lacan from a debt owed to the hysterical structure at the beginning of psychoanalysis and the turbulence of transference love. He proposes that the hysteric dreams of a desire that would be born of love, and in returning to this desire of the hysteric, he readdresses what Freud and Lacan have reiterated: that transference love is not a true love but also not a repetition.[11] To this, Safouan adds his own question: Is this "because what is at play is the very truth of love?"[12] This question invites us to reconsider the transference as the vehicle of desire and jouissance in analyses, its relation to the desire of the analyst, and its destiny in the school after the end of the analysis.

My transference to Safouan was evoked through the writings of the volume of the *Papers of the Freudian School of Melbourne* mentioned earlier which I found in a little bookshop in London near the Freud Museum. This address of an otherness in my transference to these writings, along with other writings, served as my entrance to the School. We are reminded of how Lacan in his seminar continuously questioned the transference that was concerned with the imaginary of his person.[13] In 1980, when he visited South America for the first time, he noted a hope that a transference evoked from his writings would act as a screen to his person and even allow an opening to an otherness, permitting that the psychoanalytic discourse continues to be questioned. Safouan was also present at this visit, a time of close proximity to Lacan's death, and he stresses that he was more interested in following his own path in working the psychoanalytic discourse than in becoming "a minister"

9 Safouan, M. (1996). Hebrew Moses, Egyptian Moses. In: *Papers of the Freudian School of Melbourne: Jacques Lacan: A Man and a* Woman, vol. 17. D. Pereira (Ed.), P. Anderson (Trans.). Melbourne: The Freudian School of Melbourne, p. 107.

10 Safouan, M. (1980 [1974]). In praise of hysteria. In: *Returning to Freud: Clinical Psychoanalysis in the School of Lacan*. S. Schneiderman (Ed. & Trans.). New Haven & London: Yale University Press, pp. 55–60.

11 Safouan, M. (1980 [1974]). In praise of hysteria, p. 60.

12 Safouan, M. (1980 [1974]). In praise of hysteria, p. 60.

13 Lacan, J. (1998 [1980]). The seminar, Paris, June 10th 1980. In: *The Papers of the Freudian School of Melbourne: Lacanian Psychoanalytic Writings the Lacanian Discourse*, vol. 19, D. Pereira (Ed.). Melbourne: The Freudian School of Melbourne, p. 13.

for the psychoanalytic cause.[14] This is a demarcation of the transference of work as it moves beyond Lacan as an ideal Other.[15] We continue to be confronted with this question of transference in relation to the transmission of psychoanalysis and how the written work may serve as a screen to the image of the person, whether it be Lacan or Safouan.

So I ask, by not having encountered the man Safouan, and in having known only his writing, am I any less Safouanian? No, because a writing is always a rewriting evoked by the transference of work. This Symposium is a response from each of our transferences to Safouan and to the way that his work has contributed to the psychoanalytic discourse that continues to be written in the Freudian School of Melbourne. This writing that is produced from an encounter with Safouan and his work also evokes a point of real in the transference for each one, as the opening to an otherness where the Other is missing.

14 MacCabe, C. (2012). Interview with Moustapha Safouan.
15 MacCabe, C. (2012). Interview with Moustapha Safouan.

Chapter 8

The politics of hysteria—Safouan and the question of power

Christiane Weller

Moustafa Safouan opens his chapter "In praise of hysteria" with the following statement: "Psychoanalysis began with hysteria, and psychoanalytic knowledge will always be worth only what our knowledge of this structure is worth."[1] He tells us that we need to 'know' the structure of hysteria in order to understand its effects on the psychoanalytic setting and on transference. But—and this is my contention in this chapter—it might also help us to understand the political. Safouan, as we know, was a psychoanalyst with a deep interest in politics. His book *Why the Arabs Are Not Free: The Politics of Writing* and his various papers on the topic are ample evidence of his political concerns.[2] And, I would say, he also saw psychoanalysis as a historically determined undertaking. The specificity of the family structure on which the functioning of Western society is based and the Oedipal logic integral to this structure, at least in psychoanalytic thought, is not immutable, according to Safouan. It depends, according to his response to an interview question by Michel Plon, on the historical situatedness of the father. The erosion of the father's position over time and the eventual failure of the fathers in the 20th century "erupted in an unimaginable manner" (*a éclaté d'une façon inimaginable*), to which the camps and the Holocaust testify.[3] With the waning of the father, the Oedipus complex as Freud understood it is also disappearing, and with it Freudian psychoanalysis. This at least is Safouan's provocation in 2017. And very clearly, he is not arguing for discarding psychoanalysis altogether, but, as he has maintained throughout his work, the Lacanian centring of language is pivotal in keeping psychoanalysis relevant. And this "language-concern" which is prevalent in Lacanian thought is also relevant for understanding the political.

1 Safouan, M. (1980 [1974]). In praise of hysteria. In: *Returning to Freud: Clinical Psychoanalysis in the School of Lacan*. S. Schneiderman (Ed. & Trans.). New Haven & London: Yale University Press, pp. 55–60, here p. 55. Published in French: Safouan, M. (1974). Eloge à l'hystérie. In: *Etudes sur l'Oedipe*. Paris: Editions du Seuil, pp. 206–213.

2 Safouan, M. (2007). *Why the Arabs Are Not Free: The Politics of Writing*. Boston, MA: Blackwell.

3 Plon, M. and Samoyault, T. (9 May 2017). Grand entretien avec Moustapha Safouan. In: *En attendant Nadeau. Journal de la littérature, des idées et des arts*. https://www.en-attendant-nadeau.fr/2017/05/09/grand-entretien-safouan/. Unpublished English translation by Tine Norregaard.

DOI: 10.4324/9781003712480-11

Before engaging with the question of the political, I would like to come back to the question of hysteria. Whether, and if so how, are the two related? What can be gained by reading the political in reference to the structure of hysteria, not as a narrow psychopathology but as a discourse structure which shapes the political sphere? In one of his Berkeley lectures, "Jouissance and the Death Drive," Safouan summarises the structure of hysteria as follows:

> The hysteric's problem is not with castration but with desire itself. The hysteric's problem is with the Other, inasmuch as he or she wants to prove to the other that he or she cannot give the object. Freud underlines the hysteric's attachment to the prehistorical creature one can never reach. She maintains desire as frustration, proving the Other's impossibility. Hysteria is an effort to keep, to guard, deprivation, and to prove the Other's impossibility to give her the object.[4]

One might say that the position of the hysteric is what keeps the political process going. The hysteric keeps the question of the impotence of the Other, or of power, alive. The notion of the so-called 'speaking truth to power' seems to capture that gesture of unmasking the master's position in discourse. In a possibly somewhat uncharitable way, I would suggest that our current obsession with identity and identity politics points to this. To tell one's own 'truth' and to mark the Other as liar is at the heart of the hysteric's approach. Safouan says it is the hysteric's "detection of the Other's lie" wherein her faith in the phallus resides.[5] And Safouan here illustrated this with a political metaphor: The phallus the hysteric wants is to be a "wanderer," never staying in one place, always being elsewhere, and thereby keeping the question of woman or the feminine alive.[6] "And this is why, wherever the hysteric goes, she brings war with her, ideological war, war of prestige, which we know has no object, but of which she makes herself the object."[7] The hysteric in Freud's, Lacan's and Safouan's writing is connected to the feminine position. While Safouan goes to some length to tell us that the hysteric is a he or she, the masculine marker at some point disappears from view. One might therefore ask whether the feminine position is better suited to question the master, the power structure, or again in the jargon of today: Is she more capable 'to speak truth to power'?

I would like to take a short detour via Freud's *Entwurf einer Psychologie*, his *Project for a Scientific Psychology*, which draws upon a case helpful in the course of understanding hysteria.[8] Safouan, in his paper "Hebrew Moses, Egyptian

4 Safouan, M. (2004). Jouissance and the death drive. In: *Literature and Psychology: 2000*, vol. 46, pp. 78–91, here p. 88.

5 Safouan, M. (1980). In praise of hysteria, p. 59.

6 Safouan, M. (1980). In praise of hysteria, p. 59.

7 Safouan, M. (1980). In praise of hysteria, p. 59.

8 Freud, S. (1999 [1895]). Entwurf einer Psychologie. In: *Gesammelte Werke. Nachtragsband*. A. Richards (Ed.). Frankfurt/M: Fischer, pp. 375–486. English translation: (1966), *Project for a Scientific Psychology*. SE I: 295–343, 347–387.

Moses," recapitulates Freud's analysis of Emma, the young girl from the *Entwurf* who develops a phobia in response to the traumatic effects of an encounter with two male shop assistants who seem to laugh at her and, by that, remind her of the sexual assault she suffered as an 8-year-old.[9] Safouan calls this, with Freud, the "first lie" or proton pseudos, which is not necessarily a memory. In the encounter with the two young men something "slips in between perception and consciousness, as if between flesh and leather [. . .] [T]his example takes on a dimension which goes far beyond the morbid phenomenon it uncovers."[10] And Safouan suggests here that it is the moment which Heidegger would call *In-der-Welt-Sein*, "Being-in-the-World," a moment which in Heidegger is linked to Angst or anxiety. This first notion, this proton pseudos, leads to a second one which pertains to the *aprés-coup*, the *Nachträglichkeit* which lends the past its traumatising effects from the perspective of the present or in its reconstruction. The third notion is, according to Safouan, the construction of a logic in Emma's narration which proposes cause and effect. Safouan calls this a false proposition "devoid of *material truth*."[11] We might say that the proton pseudos, or this 'first error,' inaugurates a logical chain which, even when it is in itself coherent, is nevertheless erroneous. In speaking about her experience, in her utterance, the subject is split between *énoncé* (what is said) and *énonciation* (saying). In the *énoncé*, something of the historical truth infiltrates, "as if traces of a first writing had been reworked and recomposed, reconstructed in a second untruthful writing."[12] This way something of the historical truth is conserved—in short, a return of the repressed. He concludes:

> Freud, then, found the centre of gravity of the subject in that reconstruction of the past in the present wherein resides, what the subject will have been (for example, a phobic) in function of, if not in opposition to, what it must be (for example, a woman).[13]

This proton pseudos, which agitates the neurotic or the hysteric, carries forward both the lie and the truth, and it directs it to the Other from which the subject seeks some sort of recognition. For Safouan, the example of Emma and the way Freud interprets her phobia based on this first lie corresponds with the idea of the primordial myth. Safouan noted that it was *Totem and Taboo* which made him a disciple of Freud and of psychoanalysis. This was the text to which he first developed a

9 Safouan, M. (1996). Hebrew Moses, Egyptian Moses. In: *Papers of the Freudian School of Melbourne*, vol. 17, pp. 107–116.

10 Safouan, M. (1996). Hebrew Moses, Egyptian Moses, p. 110.

11 Safouan, M. (1996). Hebrew Moses, Egyptian Moses, p. 111.

12 Safouan, M. (1996). Hebrew Moses, Egyptian Moses, p. 111. Jocelyn Benoist explores Freud's notion of *historical truth* as he developed it in reference to religion (cf. Benoist, J. (8 May 2017). Freud's 'historical truth' revisited. In: *Research in Psychoanalysis* [Online], 23: 2017/1. https://www.cairn.info/revue-research-in-psychoanalysis-2017-1-page-37.htm.

13 Safouan, M. (1996). Hebrew Moses, Egyptian Moses, p. 111.

transference—and not, as he notes, to Freud's last text, *Moses and Monotheism*.[14] It is the parricide on which the law is founded which interested Safouan, or which he, while perfectly aware of Freud's deliberate construction of an origin myth—which means, aware of Freud's lie—finds the *Totem and Taboo* narrative much more compelling or 'true' than the idea of Moses becoming the foreign leader of a tribe of nomadic people. The Moses narrative was something he found completely unbelievable or "unsound."[15] But what Safouan nevertheless acknowledges is the need for the theorist Freud to adhere to the scientific principle, namely that of cause and effect. Freud's historicisations serve exactly that function.

I would like to suggest that Safouan takes this sudden recognition of and transference to the myth of the parricide and the initial disbelief in Moses as the liberator and lawgiver as the basis of his own political theorisations. The transference to the story of the parricide makes him an analysand, so to speak, and the consideration of the function of the law, an analyst. However, he of course arrives at this by way of language and by way of his discovery of Lacan. Freud's Oedipus is displaced by Lacan's definition of "desire as the desire of the Other and by making the Other a place of language, of which the mother is the first to occupy the place" (*le désir par le désir de l'Autre et en faisant de l'Autre un lieu du langage, dont la mère est la première à occuper la place*).[16] Safouan suggests that the mythical identification with the father and the dawning of the Oedipus complex are not predicated on a passive or feminine attitude but, on the contrary, on one which Freud called "typically masculine (*exquisit männlich*)."[17] Which brings us back to the hysteric and the undermining of the Other or Master and with this to the question of law.

Safouan writes about the hysteric's relationship to the law, here a particular form of the law, as follows. This law is

> presented as a demand or commandment, [a] source of a luring, which consists in *the law's appearing to be born out of the mouth of the one who proffers it* as a law that the will of the other imposes or wants to impose and not as a law to which the other is submitted.[18]
>
> (italics in the original)

The hysteric, according to Safouan, wants to be a lawmaker based on the erroneous belief that there is an "Author of the Law."[19]

At this point, Lacan's four discourses will help to clarify the hysteric's address. We might recall that the discourse of the hysteric rotates the discourse of the master

14 Safouan, M. (1996). Hebrew Moses, Egyptian Moses, p. 108.
15 Safouan, M. (1996). Hebrew Moses, Egyptian Moses, p. 109.
16 Plon, M. et al. Unpublished English translation by Tine Norregaard.
17 Safouan, M. (1996). *Hebrew Moses, Egyptian Moses*, p. 115.
18 Safouan, M. (1980). In praise of hysteria, p. 56.
19 Safouan, M. (1980). In praise of hysteria, p. 56.

to the next quarter position. If the master discourse locates the S1 in the first position, the position of the agent, the S1 is here undercut by the barred S ($), by the knowledge of a split. In the discourse of the hysteric, the barred subject ($) now moves into the position of agent, addressing itself to the master signifier, the S1. Knowledge now moves into the position of production; and in the last position, the position of truth, we find surplus enjoyment. Lacan writes that at the level of the hysteric's discourse, "we see this dominant [that which is in the first position] appear in the form of a symptom," and he says something which he feels is true for "our own time," namely that "the law is being called into question as a symptom."[20,21]

To think about the hysteric's discourse in terms of politics is of course not new. Mia Kager, a contributor to the publications of The New Viennese Group, believes that Lacan's de-centering of the subject is the premise of the political and that it manifests itself most prominently in the discourse of the hysteric, since she repeatedly and poignantly addresses the master and asks about his legitimation. The political subject, Kager suggests, is subjugated; this is what makes it a political subject. This subjugation, this barring of the subject, is part and parcel of the act of speaking or of being implicated by the discourse of the Other. Kager refers to Derrida's idea, that the foundational paradox of the polis or the political community functions as follows: When the polis formulates itself as community, it is already in existence. That means society has already carried out the act of foundation when it eventually gets to found itself. The power of, for example, democracy is therefore determined not by its fulfilment but by its promise. It is at the same time symbolic and imaginary. While we might not be political in the way that we are political activists, we are political subjects since we are subjugated by the politics of the law(s) of language.[22] Signification is the only possibility to recognise one another as subjects or the other as subject. Kager, continuing this train of thought, suggests that the lack inscribed into the relationship of promise in reference to the other opens the possibility of desire. She states that it is desire for the desire of the other rather than recognition by the other which motivates the discourse of the hysteric and, for that matter, the political discourse.[23] The hysteric's question is addressed to this other. The S2 in the four discourses with its point of departure in the discourse of the master can be understood as the political community per se, determined

20 Lacan, J. (2007). *The Other Side of Psychoanalysis: The Seminar of Jacques Lacan: Book XVII*. R. Grigg (Trans.). New York & London: W. W. Norton & Company, p. 43.

21 Lacan, J. (2007). *The Other Side of Psychoanalysis*, p. 43.

22 Cf. Kager, M. (2013). Die Entstehung des Lacan'schen Subjekts im Diskurs der Hysterikerin. In: *Lacan 4D. Zu den vier Diskursen in Lacans Seminar XVII*. I. Gurschler, S. Ivády and A. Wald (Eds.). Wien & Berlin: Turia + Kant, pp. 144–145.

23 The questioning of the law and the destabilisation of the lawgiver in the context of the Arab world is somewhat more complicated, since it risks the annihilation of the doubter, or the hysteric for that matter, which means the idea of the 'desire for the desire of the other' within the political realm of the Arab world needs to be qualified further.

by way of the S1, the master signifier, and at the same time legitimised by its subjugation through the law and the symbolic order. The continuous and insistent questioning of the master and the master's discourse or the S1 by the hysteric suggests that she is not prepared to completely forego her attempt of *Ich-Setzung* ("self-positioning"); that something resists, something which keeps her alienated from the symbolic.[24] The hysteric doubts that the others are what they pretend to be, and she fears that she is what the other makes of her. This keeps on agitating her and her address to the master.

Slavoj Zizek attributes the capacity to undercut the master's position not only to the hysteric discourse but also to the university discourse. Both of them therefore shape the political interaction. As university discourse, it is "the expert-rule of bureaucracy that culminates in the biopolitics of reducing the population to a collection of *homo sacer*" and the hysteric discourse that culminates in "the explosion of the hysterical capitalist subjectivity that reproduces itself through permanent self-revolutionizing, through the integration of the excess into the 'normal' functioning of the social link."[25,26] These are for Zizek the "two faces of modernity": "total administration and capitalist-individualist dynamics."[27] Both Kager and particularly Zizek are concerned with modern (Western) states or democracies, which means systems where the pre-modern master has been replaced by a master already relativised by a state of law and bound by enlightened social contracts, a power structure which can be moved and subverted by the hysteric's claim, one which needs to be continuously re-negotiated. For Safouan, Western democracies present a point of departure from which to explore despotism in the Arab world. Democracies are complicated in as much as they instigate the questioning of the ruler, which means departing from "the quasi natural division between ruler and the ruled."[28] The relativisation of the (ideal) father and the incorporation of the mother (by way of the mother tongue) is at the heart of the Western democratic project.

24 Kager, M. (2013). Die Entstehung des Lacan'schen Subjekts im Diskurs der Hysterikerin, p. 152.

25 The term *homo sacer* derives from Roman law, where the 'sacred man' is at the same time the 'accursed man,' an outsider to the community and outside the law. The *homo sacer* cannot be sacrificed, while at the same time he can be killed without any repercussions for the perpetrator. Giorgio Agamben develops the category of the *homo sacer* in reference to both the biopolitics of the camps (the inmates are without rights; they are outside of the law) (cf. Agamben, G. (1998). *Homo Sacer. Sovereign Power and Bare Life*. Stanford: Stanford University Press), and in extension, we could also include the sovereign, who is also outside or above the law. In his recent work, Agamben detects the category of the *homo sacer* in the context of the pandemic, i.e. the state creating the ruse or lie (of a pandemic) which demands the widespread abolition of human rights (cf. Agamben, G. (2021). *Where Are We Now? The Epidemic as Politics*. Lanham, MA: Rowman & Littlefield.). This rather controversial idea, which buys into current conspiracy theories, however, charges modern Western states with a kind of despotism not dissimilar to what Safouan has in mind when he analyses the despotism of the Arab states.

26 Zizek, S. *Jacques Lacan's Four Discourses*. https://www.lacan.com/zizfour.htm.

27 Zizek, S. *Jacques Lacan's Four Discourses*.

28 Safouan, M. (2007). *Why the Arabs Are Not Free: The Politics of Writing*, p. 8.

The question for Safouan is how a democratic regime can ever come into being and what makes voluntary servitude and despotism so attractive.

In the final part of my chapter, I would like to refocus on Safouan and what he does with his sketch of the political discourse when reading the Arab world. This inevitably also entails a questioning of the applicability of the Oedipal structure to the position of the Arab subject. Can the familial structure which enables the Oedipal logic to function be applied to a non-Western context? The Oedipal structure which allows for the law to both function and be questioned is predicated on a dialectic, on the interchangeability between master and slave, where one could in principle ascend or descend to the position of the other. This functioning dialectic is, according to Safouan, a "purely European phenomenon."[29] Safouan locates the beginning of this shift in the high Middle Ages (mid-11th century to the mid-13th century), as a developing secularity which allows for the relativisation of power. Integral to this increasing secularity is what Safouan calls a creative transmission in contrast to a fixed transmission. The founding of the universities in medieval Europe not by the church or the state but by the stakeholders or students themselves created a different writing which was not bound by the doctrines of the church. Free thought, for Safouan, has to do with the use of language or with the way language is conscripted to certain causes. The European Middle Ages usher in a development which is, for example, continued in Luther's Reformation as well as the Enlightenment period. Creative transmission could also be seen as a kind of transgression, albeit one which is tolerated since the law is conceived of as neither divine nor absolute. To get to this—what we might call with Safouan "creative transgression"—we need to understand how he arrived there. Safouan locates this first step in the move from the primordial father to the Oedipal configuration. However, in this first move, the so-called father figure in possession of the mother and as lawgiver within the logic of Oedipus is at the same time the father ideal or "ideal ego," according to Safouan. An identification is therefore at the same time a transgression.[30] And he says in his paper "Transgression and the act of government" that imaginary transgression, which "amounts to an imaginary negation of the primordial privation," proceeds to real transgression. Here, the subject sacrificing him- or herself in His name or out of His love can become the killer or the terrorist.[31] This father figure exercises his power over the individual and the group, infantilising both in making them accept their "voluntary servitude."[32] Safouan refers here to Etienne de La Boétie's *Discours de la servitude volontaire*, which was written in approximately 1552/53 (published in 1577) and which argued for civil disobedience. However, this identification/transgression with and against the father figure

29 Safouan, M. (1994). Two modes of transmission: Creative and fixed. In: *Critical Quarterly*, vol. 36, no. 2, pp. 3–12, here p. 3.

30 Safouan, M. (2005). Transgression and the act of government. In: *Critical Quarterly*, vol. 47, no. 3, pp. 12–16, here p. 13.

31 Cf. Safouan, M. (2005). Transgression and the act of government, p. 13.

32 Safouan, M. (2005). Transgression and the act of government, p. 13.

can play out in two ways. On one hand, it can become fixed, and I would say fossilised, in what Safouan calls the logic of the Monarch. The Monarch can be everything, from the king of archaic states to the modern Islamic state. In his paper "Political authority in the Middle East," a response to 9/11, Safouan suggests that the Monarch's authority is legitimated not by the people but by religion.[33] That means this kind of Monarch or government, or the One, is making it impossible for its subjects to even think of themselves as "being united in order to defend a common interest."[34] Only the Monarch or the One has, as it were, access to the truth via his authority based on the divine. This exclusive relation between the Monarch and God or religion, which refuses any dialectic engagement with his/her subjects, is stabilised in a writing. Safouan recalls Claude Lévi-Strauss's observation in *Triste Tropiques*, that only the development of writing makes the emergence of states and state power possible. But, and this is I think the important contribution by Safouan, a writing can fossilise or negotiate truth claims. In the case of the Middle East, Safouan suggests, the writing or the language used by the Monarch (i.e. the state's administration, etc.) had prevented it from being accessed by the common people. The vernacular, for example in Egypt, had never been "adopted as the written language of administration and culture."[35] The classical Arabic taught at school and connected to the Koran, but not spoken in the community, maintains the schism between the Monarch and his/her subjects. Truth or a truth claim is therefore always only possible with reference to a writing which draws its legitimacy from the sphere of the sacred. This might be compared to the pharaoh who inscribed his obelisk with a writing which could not be understood by his subjects but which announced the unquestioned position, legitimacy and power of the One. Linguistic humanism, which enabled the European cultures to force power into dialogue with the people (as we can see in Dante's use of Italian as a literary language or Luther's bible translation into German) and negotiate notions of truth, is, according to Safouan, made impossible by the language policies in the Middle East, which continue to serve an absolute claim to truth and power.[36] Safouan remarks that the use of the vernacular or the mother tongue, replacing the "dead" Latin, introduces the mother or the body of the mother into the body politics. The use and status of this mother tongue are not unequivocal, since they keep alive the opposition or the destabilisation of the "grammatical" language of the father. Applied to the Arab world, the insistence of maintaining the universal classical Arabic (a "dead" language according to Safouan) as the language of the university, bureaucracy and the sovereign negates difference and excludes the mother-tongue or Lalangue. This in turn disallows the animating reverberation of Lalangue in the body of the speaker,

33 Cf. Safouan, M. (2003). Political authority in the Middle East. In: *Critical Quarterly*, vol. 45, nos. 1–2, pp. 113–119, here p. 113.
34 Safouan, M. (2003). Political authority in the Middle East, p. 114.
35 Safouan, M. (2003). Political authority in the Middle East, p. 116.
36 Cf. Safouan, M. (2007). *Why the Arabs Are Not Free: The Politics of Writing*, p. 94.

from which desire and opposition might be animated. Safouan's critique of the Arab states is blunt: They rely on "repression and corruption" keeping millions in a "state of servitude."[37] A first step of democratisation is, according to Safouan, linked to the accepted use of the vernacular languages within the universities, the administrations and within poetry and literature.

When Martin Luther addresses the Diet of Worms to defend his call for a reformation of the church, he resorts to his own truth, a civil disobedience in the face of a possible death sentence. He asserts his right to speak "truth to power," or to hystericise his position to call into question the position of the master.[38] This is political activism, which Safouan says that Lacan eventually fell victim to when he tried to assert his power and authority in the face of internal resistance within his School. But what about Safouan himself? Is his critique of the theocratic governments of the Middle East and his demand for an enlightened Arab culture a necessary hysterisation of his position, and how does this impact on his position as an analyst? We might also ask what it means in a Western, capitalist democracy to critique state power today and how one can hystericise one's own position in order to do so.

I would like to finish with a few remarks on a curious case in recent Australian politics. The now-former prime minister of Australia, Scott Morrison, a devout Christian and member of a Pentecostal church, secretly assumed altogether five ministries despite those being held by apparently trusted members of the government. Neither the public nor the respective ministers, bar one, were informed about these appointments, which means that almost everyone except the prime minister operated without any knowledge of the clandestine power grab.[39] One might say that the prime minister installed himself into the position of the Monarch, communicating nothing to 'his' subjects, or more precisely, not having the symbolic resonance chamber. He might have delighted in the knowledge that he had successfully bypassed the conventions of a democratic state and made himself into a quasi-religious leader who was called upon by a higher power.[40] Later, he claimed that while he had to seize these powers to defend against the COVID-19 pandemic, he supposedly never used or misused them. He rather surprisingly completely misunderstood the conventions of a modern democracy, or the principles of the Reformation and the Enlightenment, for that matter. On the face of it, this looked like the move of an autocrat, better suited to someone who would establish his position

37 Safouan, M. (2007). *Why the Arabs Are Not Free: The Politics of Writing*, p. 92.

38 Luther's most famous words *Hier stehe ich. Ich kann nicht anders* ("Here I stand, I can do no other"), supposedly spoken at the Diet of Worms in 1521, only appeared in the written report sometime later. However, they forever mark the idea that the political activist needs to refer to and testify with his body.

39 The exception was Greg Hunt, who held the health portfolio.

40 In her book *Bulldozed*, Niki Savva recalls the observation of a prominent liberal that Morrison felt he was ordained by God (Savva, N. (2022). *Bulldozed. Scott Morrison's Fall and Anthony Albanese's Rise*. Melbourne & London: Scribe, p. 19).

within a theocratic or totalitarian system, a move also better suited to a politician like Donald Trump. However, the hubris shown by Morrison made him a figure of ridicule when finally exposed. The hysterical discourse, but possibly also the university discourse—i.e. the secular administration or bureaucracy—worked in so far as nobody was convincingly able or willing to condone such autocratic behaviour.[41] Destabilising the power Morrison had invested in himself was a non-event in so far as the model of the Monarch had clearly no currency in Australia. The glance of disdain given him by the activist and 2021 Australian of the Year, Grace Tame, during a short address to the press, marked the hollowness of Morrison's claim to power. The evocation of being ordained by the One, or the reference to a historical truth which could give legitimacy to his behaviour, fell flat in a thoroughly secular society which had become highly suspicious of such 'truth' claims, unmasking them as delusional. Could one therefore say that the hysteric discourse which demotes the master for his refusal to deliver on the promise of democracy has become the ubiquitous discourse of today, relying not only on a parliamentarian opposition but utilising and amplifying individual protests, accusations or simply disdain? And if so, what about the category of the feminine itself, traditionally so intertwined with the discourse of hysteria? Can the feminine be rewritten or rephrased in light of the political discourse, as we have outlined? Could the hysteric's quest for the 'true' woman within this political arena disappear? How can we conceptualise this hysteria without a (bodily) pathology? Hysteria according to this reading would become the political gesture which keeps the process of stabilising and destabilising power going.

41 As Zizek has it (cf. Zizek, S. *Jacques Lacan's Four Discourses*).

Chapter 9

Why the subject is not free?

Michael Gerard Plastow

Moustapha Safouan, towards the end of his career, collected some essays into a book that was first published in English under the title *Why Are the Arabs Not Free? The Politics of Writing*. The following year, a new version was produced in French, and here, Safouan's "Preface to the French Translation" curiously misquotes the title of the original English version as, *Why the Arabs are not Free?* producing the ambiguity of a statement and a question, an ambiguity that I wish to preserve here.[1] The title in French is slightly different and is no longer in fact a question at all and translates as *Why the Arab World Is Not Free* (no question mark): *The Politics of Writing and Religious Terrorism*. Here, I would like to draw upon Safouan's thesis by endeavouring to subtract the reference to politics, to the polis, in order to examine—as in a silhouette—what this book might convey regarding the subject in psychoanalysis, specifically in relation to the question of freedom and writing. What is the place of freedom for the subject in psychoanalysis, or is this something that is just taken from the field of the political? Already in the different versions of the title, there is an equivocation between the Arab world and the Arab, that is, between the political and the particular.

But let us first attempt to give a brief account of Safouan's thesis in this book: Since the beginning of history, political power in the Middle East has always drawn its legitimacy from religion. This goes together with the fact that written language was made sacred, to the detriment of the everyday spoken language, for the purposes of prestige and exploitation. The language of learning in Arab nations is classical Arabic, which is the language of the Koran, that is, the language not just of the time of the Prophet but of the particular tribe and locality from which he came. Safouan tells us that this language is as different to the different modalities of Arabic that are spoken across the Arab world as they are to each other. "The people are isolated from the field of thought by the confinement of writing in a classical language,"[2] he puts forward, and they are subject to states—including

1 Safouan, M. (2008). *Pourquoi le monde arabe n'est pas libre: Politique de l'écriture et terrorisme religieux*. Paris: Denoël, p. 11 [The translation is my own, as are all that follow. MGP].
2 Safouan, M. (2008). *Pourquoi le monde arabe n'est pas libre*, p. 138.

DOI: 10.4324/9781003712480-12

the Islamic State—that "usurped that attribute of God of being he who has the final knowledge and interpretation."[3] Safouan's own efforts to remedy the poor position in which the vernacular language is held has been in part to translate texts, in particular Shakespeare's *Othello*, into demotic Egyptian Arabic. By his own admission, the effects of such efforts have been derisory, little read and poorly staged. For Safouan, "translation into Arabic should not follow a so-called ideal of arabisation; quite the contrary, translation consists of utilising language in order to liberate us from the limits that language itself imposes on us."[4] Here translation, a work of writing, is put forward as an activity that can be used in the promotion of freedom from the enslavement by language.

Safouan asserts that the first movements towards freedom in Europe resulted, at least in part, in the privileging of the "mother tongue," which had hitherto been banned from being taught, to the benefit of what Dante called the "grammatical language,"[5] Latin in his case. Safouan cites Dante, who wrote in *De Vulgari Eloquentia* that "of these two languages, the vulgar is the most noble."[6] Safouan claims that this is, "the declaration of independence"[7] of European languages, partially explaining the fact that Dante's writing of his *Divine Comedy* in vulgar Tuscan had such a determining effect on the Italian language such as we know it today.

Safouan begins his book by citing a text that dates from 1530 by a French writer, Estienne de la Boétie, which is called *Discourse on Voluntary Servitude*.[8] De la Boétie was associated with a group of French Renaissance writers known as La Pléiade, who, like Safouan in regard to Arabic, privileged vernacular French. La Boétie's tract was taken up during periods of political agitation and is known by revolutionary groups as *Contre l'un, Against the One*. La Boétie's question was, "how is it that one man, the monarch, can reduce millions of subjects into slavery?" a question that would have a big impact on Moustapha Safouan with his personal history of dictatorships in both Egypt and the Arab world at large. He contrasts this to the separation of powers in modern European democracies, of which he holds the American Constitution as their model, and in particular the "First Amendment [. . .] ratified in 1791, which stipulates that Congress would not ratify any law forbidding the free exercise of religious beliefs, limiting freedom of speech, or that of the press,"[9] and so on.

But from the democratic, we might choose to separate out the demotic, or vernacular language, from the -cratic, in other words, the question of power. La Boétie himself begins with an epigraph from Homer's *Iliad*, citing Ulysses rousing the

3 Safouan, M. (2008). *Pourquoi le monde arabe n'est pas libre*, p. 138.
4 Safouan, M. (2008). *Pourquoi le monde arabe n'est pas libre*, p. 88.
5 Safouan, M. (2008). *Pourquoi le monde arabe n'est pas libre*, p. 27.
6 Safouan, M. (2008). *Pourquoi le monde arabe n'est pas libre*, p. 81.
7 Safouan, M. (2008). *Pourquoi le monde arabe n'est pas libre*, p. 81.
8 Estienne de la Boétie. *La Servitude Volontaire*. https://www.gutenberg.org/files/62051/62051-h/62051-h.htm.
9 Safouan, M. (2008). *Pourquoi le monde arabe n'est pas libre*, p. 23.

Greek forces, uttering the following words: "I see no good in having several lords; let one alone be master, let one alone be king."[10]

La Boétie notes that Ulysses says these words in public, and at that moment, he may have been obliged to say this in order to quell a mutiny in the army that was being assembled to fight the Trojans, and in his opinion chooses language to meet an emergency rather than in order to speak the truth. Thus in this instance, La Boétie differentiates speech from truth. Here, we might perceive the position of the hysteric: We find a *proton pseudos*, a first lie, at the heart of hysterical discourse, just like all writing relies on a false start, a false premise from which a true conclusion may be derived.

Let us then endeavour to differentiate what we might call the *Homo politicus*, the being of the polis, from the singular subject. And in case anyone might consider this term politically incorrect, we clarify that we are using *homo*—as Lacan does—to signify 'same': this homo is equal under the law of the land, and has the same rights to vote. This is the Latin subjectus: a subject that refers to the being subjected, who submits to the state, to the monarch or the dictator. The other form of subject from Latin is the subjectum, conveying the sense of something that is put underneath: a material substratum. In this way, we might separate out the *Homo politicus* from another species that we can designate as the *Heteros atopicus*, the subject of Otherness of no fixed address, marked by its singularity, by the single stroke of *Einzigkeit*, of singularity.

For Safouan, Islam labours under the notion that all powers are concentrated in the hands of the sultan, emir or caliph, the latter literally signifying successor. That is, the caliph is the successor of the Prophet and therefore the representative of God on earth. For the subject, though, specifically the psychoanalytic subject, there is no possibility of being free of the Other. As Lacan stated, *Y a d'l'un*, "There is of the one," which is inescapable. Lacan insists that this "of the One" is the master signifier, a non-contingent signifier, then, rather than an embodied master or monarch.

Safouan states that the politics of oneness—and here this is a oneness of unity, that is, an *Einheit*—consists in banning the mother tongue from schools, as indeed the colonists did with indigenous peoples in this country. In this way, the "grammatical language" retains its place of privilege. For Safouan, then, in ancient cultures—as well as for despotic modern cultures—"the mother tongue . . . was considered as a popular idiom, unsuitable for expressing elevated ideas."[11] By the mother tongue being devalued in this way, "it becomes devalued in the eyes of the people themselves, and prevents them from thinking of a freedom that they do not merit, and which doesn't suit them."[12] Nonetheless, this mother tongue "is the

10 *Oὐκ ἀγαθον πολυκοιρανιη εἱς κοιρανος ἐστω Εἱς βασιλευς*. Estienne de la Boétie, *La Servitude Volontaire*.

11 Safouan, M. (2008). *Pourquoi le monde arabe n'est pas libre*, p. 25.

12 Safouan, M. (2008). *Pourquoi le monde arabe n'est pas libre*, p. 26.

language that the people learn in the cradle and in which they pass their lives, from birth to death."[13]

It is at this point that we need to separate out the mother tongue in its significance to the political subject from something that Lacan refers to as lalangue and its importance for the singular subject. Lacan introduces this—he says—as a slip of the tongue when making a reference to the dictionary of philosophy by Lalande, a philosopher who was an acquaintance of Safouan. Lalangue emerges as a formation of the unconscious, a homophony and alliteration of Lalande and lalangue, but also of *lallation*: lallation also in English. Lallation is the babbling of the *infans*, taking part in the joy of jabbering, the delight of lallation. But the babbling of the babe endeavours to reach up to the mother's murmurs, a babble that endeavours to construct the oneness of a Tower of Babel in order to reach and to share the mother's tongue. However, as we know, this tower is doomed to collapse as the subject's language. Lalangue inexorably tears away from that of the mother.

In his book *Lacaniana*, Safouan notes that lalangue refers to a language that is singular for each one, transmitted by this first Other that was their mother. Safouan defines it in the following way:

> [I]t is not just a question of the mother tongue, understood as that which the mother spoke, French, English, et cetera, but rather that of lalangue in which the subject was from the beginning immersed, of that singular one of this mother, with the words that were proper to her, her inventions, her funny ways, and from the beginning a signifying equivocation.[14]

Thus, if lalangue is not just the mother tongue, it is then the singular way in which each subject is marked by the mother tongue, this fleshy organ by which they are stroked. And this singularity—the oneness of the single stroke or *Einzigkeit*—is also the singularity that may emerge from an analysis. Later, Safouan tells us that the preponderant place in the formation of lalangue is that attributed to the voice: the invocatory object.[15]

What of the place of writing, which is such an important signifier in Safouan's book? Safouan himself was someone who felt the necessity to write, of writing what is impossible to say. He argues that since ancient times, writing has been used as a weapon of political oppression, particularly of illiterate and conquered peoples. "From its first appearance," he states, "writing has taken the form of revealed truth. [. . .] Its creation, like the creation of the world itself, was always attributed to a God."[16] It was only in ancient Athens that writing was no longer a monopoly

13 Safouan, M. (2008). *Pourquoi le monde arabe n'est pas libre*, p. 79.

14 Safouan, M. (2005). *Lacaniana: Les séminaires de Jacques Lacan 1964–1979*. Paris: Fayard, p. 282.

15 Safouan, M. (2005). *Lacaniana*, p. 387.

16 Safouan, M. (2008). *Pourquoi le monde arabe n'est pas libre*, p. 111.

in the hands of a certain category of the population. Only at that time, according to Safouan, "It became possible to think of the Law (nomos), not as something revealed, but something relative, that depended on the will of the people." Hence, for Safouan, the significance of Plato's critique was to withhold from writing its sacred character. Thus, for the first time in human history, Plato extricated the notion of rationality from any connection with belief. But perhaps here, there is a conflation of the question of the sacred with that of belief, something we might need to tease out.

This again may be where we might distinguish the political being from the subject. The being of the polis is one for whom belief predominates, as Freud demonstrates in his *Group Psychology and the Analysis of the Ego* in reference to the church and the army, both social institutions, dominated by a leader, a *Führer*. It is in these institutions that belief is required, belief in the institution and belief in the leader. Nothing is sacred in politics. The political being could say, for instance, "This is a victory for the true believers, the people who in difficult times have kept the faith and to the Australian people going through hard times—it makes their act of faith all that much greater."[17] Faith and belief are the hallmarks here. Safouan notes that the founding priority of belief is that of the symbolic order. Thus the secret of authority is the deception of embodying the symbolic order, the place of transcendence, the third place outside that of the narcissistic relation based on similarity.

If Plato extricated the notion of rationality and belief from writing, surely he did not remove from writing its sacred nature. According to Walter Benjamin, the mark of all great texts is their very untranslatability. Of these, he comments that they "contain their potential translation between the lines."[18] Benjamin remarks that it is in the Holy Writ alone that meaning has ceased to be the watershed for the flow of language and of revelation: It is this that vouchsafes language from the endless slippage of meaning, of interpretation. It is this very untranslatability that distinguishes the sacredness of a text, whether it is Holy Writ or not. This sacredness has traditionally been attributed to God, and we understand sacred here as pertaining to a text that does not lend itself to translation, including psychoanalytic texts, literature, and especially poetry. Safouan stresses that the Koran is the word of God, but in written form. And God's word, in the Jewish tradition, is both unpronounceable and unutterable, hence is limited to writing. It is the very sacredness of the text that makes it not contingent, unnegotiable, unlike the political deal.

What of freedom, then, in psychoanalysis? Lacan was rather sceptical of the notion of freedom: "Liberty, Equality, Fraternity, for example, that's indecent," he said, criticising the political notion of freedom that arose out of the student protests

17 Paul Keating. https://speakola.com/political/paul-keating-sweetest-victory-1993.

18 Benjamin, W. (1999). (Edited and with an Introduction by Hannah Arendt). The task of the translator. In: *Illuminations*. H. Zorn (Trans.). London: Pimlico, p. 82.

of May 1968.[19] And further still, as he put to the students at Vincennes University, "What you aspire to as revolutionaries, is to have a master. You will have one."[20] So for Lacan, the notion of political freedom cannot be dissociated from the discourses in which the subject finds itself, in this case the discourse of the master. But whilst politics may be conducted on a more or, as Safouan points out, less ethical basis, psychoanalysis is by its very nature an ethical pursuit: the ethics of the unconscious.

Freedom, for Kant, is the freedom to make, whilst at the same time obeying, universal law. But this universal law is devoid of any contingency, of moral law or of the superego. It is this same lack of contingency that we have discussed in relation to what is construed in holy writ as God, the source of its sanctity. In psychoanalysis, the object is non-contingent. It is the object in so far as it is no longer the breast as object of satisfaction nor the faeces as object of exchange nor even the scopic object in the field of fantasy. To take up something that we isolated earlier, this object can only be the voice or invocatory object in so far as it does not correspond to any sensible object and is not representable as such. It is this which is the object of psychoanalysis and which allows the freedom to create or to give things new form, which Freud said is the very function of the unconscious. If for the analysand this is free association, for the analyst, it is the evenly suspended attention. In the transference, it is the analyst who is the contingent object, the object to be satisfied, exchanged or even fantasised, but an object to be dispensed with when the analysis reaches its term.

Thus the freedom—to take up Safouan's term from the title of this book—in psychoanalysis is not a freedom to do whatever one chooses: It is rather a constraint upon the subject to unceasingly endeavour to liberate oneself from the signifiers, meanings and contingent objects in which one is caught in order to destroy these so that one can continue to create and invent. This is also the politics of writing in so far as writing is the concrete support of the signifier. Writing is the necessary task of endeavouring to reach an impossible, in this case of addressing the polis, the Other, in order to continue to erode fixed meanings and presuppositions, to thereby be able to invent.

19 Lacan, J. (2013 [1971–1972]). *The Knowledge of the Psychoanalyst/Le Savoir du Psychanalyste* (Bilingual edition). Paris: Association Lacanienne Internationale (Non-commercial publication), p. 143.

20 Lacan, J. (1991). *Le Séminaire livre XVII: L'Envers de la psychanalyse*. Paris: Seuil, p. 239.

Chapter 10

For the love of Safouan

Transference and identification in the Freudian school

David Pereira

Preparing for this Symposium in honour of Moustapha Safouan once again gave me cause to pose the question of what moves one to write a paper? Particularly striking on this occasion was that—not unlike the experience of an analysis—it allows a way of engaging with what haunts me, the reminiscences from which I suffer. The hope being to endeavour to situate oneself differently with respect to the knowledge, the history we are inhabited by and which haunts us.

So today, we are paying our respects to Moustapha Safouan, whose death marks a particular moment in the history of psychoanalysis. Although I am not averse to the term 'death,' on this occasion, I am nonetheless inclined to take it as a 'passing' and to try and engage with what passes to us.

To begin with, two citations from works of Safouan which I hope form an apt preface to what I plan to try and work in this chapter.

> [I]n order to transform what you learn into knowledge, you have to transmit the lesson of your experience.[1]
>
> But the transference, as we know, carries the best and the worst.[2]

In this context, then, I will offer you, for better or for worse, something of my own experience—the lesson of my experience—as it pertains to the history of my own formation in psychoanalysis, intersected as it was by meeting Safouan in Melbourne on two occasions.

This writing, driven by a haunting, will proceed by way of a series of reminiscences, and to this extent, it engages in a certain hysterical modality. These reminiscences are not always welcomed by me but are nonetheless important in assisting in a navigation of the complex path of a transmission between transference and identification, perennially important parameters, inevitably problematic within any

1 Safouan, M. (1990). On supervision. In: *Papers of the Freudian School of Melbourne*, vol. 11, O. Zentner (Ed.), pp. 167–177. The Freudian School of Melbourne.
2 Safouan, M. (1984). Jacques Lacan and the training of analysts. In: *Papers of the Freudian School of Melbourne*, vol. 5, O. Zentner (Ed.), pp. 157–221. The Freudian School of Melbourne.

DOI: 10.4324/9781003712480-13

school of psychoanalysis engaged in the formation of analysts. Whilst what I will share with you today passes very close to what may seem confessional, it does not proceed with any hope of absolution. Rather, only of continuing to afford me the possibility of mis-taking my errors, making mistakes out of my errors.

Before proceeding any further, however, I need to clarify something concerning an uncomfortable presumption carried in my title, "For the love of Safouan," by this rather heavy word, "love." There is a clear touch of mimicry to the title, even if dignified by reference to identification.

Derrida's homage to Lacan in 1990, published as "For the love of Lacan," in playing no small part in the fabrication of my own title, adds further to the level of presumption.[3] Derrida's text, and I am not going to do it justice here, essentially speaks of this love as a numerable or countable series of *missed* encounters. In so doing, he subtracts something from the counting of the ways of love introduced in *Sonnet 43* of Elizabeth Barrett Browning's "How do I love thee? Let me *count* the ways."[4] The inevitability of a missed encounter subtracts from the possibility of counting in love.

For Derrida—I would say following Lacan and his love of Lacan—this is typical of the conditions under which we can speak of love. As specifically concerns his relationship with Lacan, his self-confessed presumptuousness is in having the right to say, "We loved each other, Lacan and I."[5] Presumptuous insofar as any amorous performative necessarily risks the presumption that, in the encounter, each counted equally; that there was or is a meeting of two "I's" in the presumptive form of a "We"; "We loved each other."

Now, my presumption is far less ambitious than Derrida's. Nonetheless, how is it possible, by what right, can I speak of love in relation to Safouan? For certain, Safouan did not know who I was. Although I had the privilege of meeting him on two occasions, is it not absurd for me to claim to know Safouan sufficiently to entertain the presumption of love?

And yet is not this very absurdity—the presumption of love in the face of the absence of a knowing—the very stuff of the cornerstone of psychoanalysis? Transference as that species of love relying upon a "not-knowing" which invites a supposing, in turn keeping an embarrassed embrace with a presumption of love.

So this phrase "for the love of Safouan" opens to the fragility of a relationship to what is known. We will return to this later in considering the formative meeting of psychoanalysis with the hysteric. For the moment, I want to return to my own formative meeting with Safouan and its influence upon my formation in psychoanalysis as affected by the vicissitudes of transference and identification.

3 Derrida, J. (1998). For the love of Lacan. In: *Resistances of Psychoanalysis*. P. Kamuf, P.-A. Brault and M. Naas (Trans.). Stanford, CA: Stanford University Press, pp. 39–69.

4 Barrett Browning, E. (1900 [1850]). How do I love thee? Let me count the ways. Sonnet 43. In: *Sonnets from the Portuguese*. Portland & Maine: Thomas B Mosher.

5 Derrida, J. (1998). For the love of Lacan, p. 42.

So a little bit of history first which will hopefully lay the ground for our praise of hysteria.

As I said a moment ago, I had the privilege of meeting Safouan—the person of Safouan—in Melbourne on two occasions. I had supposed the first of these encounters to be in 1984 at the consulting rooms of María-Inés Rotmiler de Zentner and Oscar Zentner. The second of these encounters was in the Department of Psychological Medicine at the then Prince Henry's Hospital on St Kilda Road in 1986.

Now, if you hear me gradually substituting the term "encounter" for "meeting," it is to the extent that I find myself unwilling to continue to entertain the further presumption that I "met" him. There was no "meeting." He was there. I was there. We were even introduced, as a kindness extended to me by María-Inés and Oscar, colleagues and friends of Safouan, who had invited him to Melbourne as a guest of the School. There was an encounter of sorts, but there was no "meeting," leaving me—a twenty-something-year-old who had not long begun an analysis—some work to do. As you will have gathered, I am still engaged in this work, still haunted by an encounter and the insistence of certain reminiscences which flow from it.

There is, however, another reason why I elect to use the term "encounter." It allows me to note that there was, in regard to the dating of these reminiscences, another mis-meeting. As evidence that transference is well and truly at play, this memory has since proved unreliable; something simply didn't add up.

The unreliability of my memory is demonstration of one irrevocable conclusion: that if something didn't add up, it is to the extent that I couldn't count. More poignantly, that *I didn't count* under the conditions—inevitably narcissistic—in which I sought to be counted, to be counted amongst the set of those whom I supposed counted.[6]

Let me try to explain.

My reminiscences, redolent with elements of transference and identification, were in error, assuming the hysterical marker of a *proton pseudos*—a first lie, a false premise. Safouan was not, in fact, in Melbourne in 1984, as I had falsely remembered or fabricated it, but in 1981—an original time in which I was not present—and then again in 1986, when I was able to attend two seminars. These somewhat pedestrian details are important.

What I had supposed to be two encounters separated by two years—making the second encounter remote to and separate from the first—were in fact two encounters within one visit in 1986. Somehow, this "two together" did not seem to command quite the same gravitas as one and then another. It didn't and still doesn't seem to count in the same way: this two-together in one visit, rather than one and then a separate other.

6 It is precisely the fact that something doesn't add up in the field of one's remembering that marks the distinction between the drift of reminiscence as prone to the error in the way one counts and a comfortable expedition of nostalgia always staying upon the well-worn and safely mapped path.

The fictional encounter of 1984, this *proton pseudos*, was a fabrication—unconscious—in order to make myself count in the second visit by insinuating myself into the origins; by *identifying* myself amongst those who counted. To count, therefore, with the support of a lazy imaginary identification, at the level of my "being," a falsified being there where I was not. The machinations of transference, through the devices of forgetting or mis-remembering, gave rise to a form of identification as a plagiarised and therefore false originality.[7]

The question I am re-opening today given by this phrase, "for the love of Safouan," is whether it becomes possible, through the agency of a love which resists its regression to an identification endorsed through emblems and insignia of "being," to count differently; to engage in a different mode of counting? To make a difference rather than seeking to *be* at the origins, seeking to *be* original.

In order to further clarify this, let's return to the scene of my first actual encounter. I remember a gentle man who smoked incessantly and drank whiskey with just a dash of water as he spoke of transference. I remember a man concretely engaged with the loves of the body, reminiscent, let's say, for it is a day to indulge our reminiscences, of the definition of medicine offered by Eryximachus in another *Symposium*, that of Plato, a definition which Lacan saw fit to appropriate for psychoanalysis, as not just a knowledge of the body as a fixed and static body of knowledge, but a knowledge of the *loves* of the body.[8] My own transference was immediate as I encountered a man who bore an uncanny resemblance to my greatly loved but somewhat remote grandfather.

Now, what bearing did this have upon the vicissitudes of identification which followed?

Firstly, I did not go on to drink whiskey and smoke cigarettes; these were not to be my poisons. I did not identify *with* Safouan. The identification *of* Safouan *with* my grandfather as an object of remote love paved the way for identifications with some who were a little more proximate, yet remote enough. Those whom I supposed to be Safouan's psychoanalytic progeny; whom I considered to be objects of Safouan's love, respect and admiration. Those whom I admired and certainly idealised. These were the ones who counted insofar as they were present at the first encounter, the first count. These were the ones whose traits I identified with.

At a superficial level, this consisted of the assumption of certain emblematic traits—playing at being the analyst—so as to bear the insignia of those whom I supposed as counting. Such is the kind of identification which Janet Malcolm amused

7 Lacan, J. (1961–1962). *The Seminar of Jacques Lacan Book IX Identification*. C. Gallagher (Trans.). Unpublished manuscript, session of 07.03.62. This error of the count speaks of the vicissitudes of identification under the sway of transference, something which was recognised by Lacan in noting that the significance of error for the subject was always discoverable as an error in his count, such that for the subject who does not count, there can be no error.

8 Plato. (1993). *The Dialogues of Plato. Vol. II, The Symposium*. R. E. Allen (Trans.). New Haven, CT: Yale University Press, p. 127.

us with in her observations of the New York Psychoanalytic Institute; amused on the condition of failing to recognise ourselves as in it up to our necks.

It was, however, more importantly, in another respect of the reduction of transference to identification, that the more corrosive poison was manufactured. A poison which reduced the possibility of a knowledge of the loves of the body—let's say the knowledge brought by hysteria to psychoanalysis—into a static, inert, readily identifiable body of knowledge. In this is encountered a certain impasse of the transference which seeks ratification, recognition and identification in relation to certain emblems and insignia of knowledge.

What was able to loosen the fixity of this plagiarised 'being-there' of identification? What was the work capable of subtracting from a false originality premised upon a one of identity which draws its sustenance from the one of unification? Two moments loom large in addressing this question.

Firstly, the event of my analysis and the absolute originality of my analyst—María-Inés Rotmiler de Zentner—who denied me orthodoxy in a sustained refusal of my demand for an ultra-orthodox, ultra-meaningful, so-called 'Lacanian' analysis. In her sustained refusal of my demand was carried a resistance to the reduction of transference to the insignias of identification. This left room, as Lacan has so exquisitely put it, for error to take flight in deception to be recovered as mistake.[9] Room to make mistakes out of my errors, as I clearly still am doing today.

Secondly, a particularly decisive encounter with Oscar Zentner in his seminar at Prince Henry's Hospital—in the same room but a few years after the second encounter with Safouan in 1986. I remember one seminar in particular, not for the piece of knowledge which I tucked under my arm and walked away with but quite the contrary. Rather, I remember the stinging sensation of being dislodged with respect to the trajectory of knowledge I was on. In response to a question posed by Oscar Zentner in that seminar, I formulated an answer—precise, cross-referenced, with no margin for error and in my best 'Lacanese.' Surely, this would earn me the longed-for recognition of my 'being'; being amongst the counted. What I did receive, however, and I remain grateful for it still today, was a slap. A slap in the form of what I remember as something like: "So? Any ape could tell me that! Tell me what *you* think."

Curiously, I heard this again in reading Derrida's *For the love of Lacan*, in his concern for the renovation of psychoanalytic curricula such that they might proceed in other than, he writes: "an apelike, orthodox and defensive manner."[10] I read this today as the possibilities of a transference producing a mode of identification—essentially hysterical—which nonetheless allows us to count differently and therefore propitiously with respect to a knowledge as not already known, not already accounted for.

9 Lacan, J. (1988). *The Seminar of Jacques Lacan: Book I. Freud's Papers on Technique 1953–1954*. J.-A. Miller (Ed.), J. Forrester (Trans.). Cambridge: Cambridge University Press, p. 273.

10 Derrida, J. (1998). For the love of Lacan, p. 60.

To remind you, then, of the citation from Safouan concerning hysteria which opens the invitation to this symposium: "Psychoanalytic knowledge will always be worth only what our knowledge of this structure is worth."[11] It is important to read this carefully, such that we don't fail to hear that it is not that psychoanalysis ends up "knowing" more about hysteria but that the encounter with hysteria produced an altered relationship to knowledge.

If history, the history given through my reminiscences replete with error, opens onto hysteria at this point, it is insofar as it valorises the very status of this 'other knowledge'—the knowledge of hysteria—brought by the fruit of error. You will recall this same fruit of error in the Garden of Eden, plucked from that tree, known—even well known—as the tree of knowledge. From the well-rooted and established tree of knowledge is dislodged the fruitful error of a sin. Such is the sinful encounter between psychoanalysis and hysteria not simply as producing more firmly rooted knowledge but as opening a protean or new *relationship* to knowledge as a sinful knowledge of the loves of the body.

From that breach in the historical can be heard rising the voice of hysteria. For me, therefore, the phrase "for the love of Safouan" is an essentially hysterical formula, a hinge point of this relationship between the historical and the hysterical, appearing at precisely that point of a *proton pseudos*, a false premise in the history. The fruit of an error ripened by love.

In this sense, the phrasing "for the love of Safouan" invites a different way of counting as much as a different relationship to knowledge. In being detached from the original, subtracted from the place of the origin, one either lazily identifies with the emblems of 'being', playing at being the analyst through plagiarising oneself into the origins with those you suppose count. Or one starts to count differently; counting through the instrumentality of a desire which, in refusing to be rationed in an identifiable being, dislocates being in the direction of a becoming. If such a becoming can allow itself any form of identification, the emblem I choose today is "for the love of Safouan."

This, for better or for worse, has been the lesson of my experience.

11 Safouan, M. (1980). In praise of hysteria, p. 55.

Part IV

Beyond organisation—real erotics of the word

Chapter 11

A slice of the word

David Pereira

> And may the torrent of love plunge into impasses! [. . .] New ways I go, a new speech comes to me.[1]

> Love plagues me.[2]

When I left the country of my birth and came to Australia as a young boy, I apparently lost a language I was said to be fluent in though it was not my mother tongue. Nonetheless, I have in my possession a Grade 3 report card from Wesley College Colombo, a piece of factual evidence—whatever credibility we may give to facts other than as the starting point for the construction of myths—that I had a fluency in Sinhalese. I have no memory of it now. More astonishing to me is that I had no memory of it from the time I set foot in Australia in 1969, the same year Neil Armstrong, so strangely, set foot on the moon in a piece of pure lunacy.

In 1969, in first setting foot on the surface of Australia, I lost any facility or capacity with a language I had comfortably inhabited up to that point in time. The thing about Sinhala was that it was for me a language of utility, a language of transaction—for addressing domestic staff and shopkeepers.

It was not that Sinhala became strange to me; it disappeared. What I have thought over the years was that I did not so much lose a language as lose a sense of utility in language, the loss of the functionality of a speech within a field of language.

In arriving to Australia, I remained essentially mute for a period of time. Why I could not speak is open to many possible interpretations. What interests me more, however, is why I subsequently spoke at all. The beginnings of speaking again were tortuous, laboured and stutteringly hesitant. There was, for me, nothing that could be taken for granted about speech and speaking.

1 Nietzsche, Friedrich. (2006). *Thus Spoke Zarathustra: A Book for All and None*. Cambridge Texts in the History of Philosophy. Cambridge: Cambridge University Press, p. 64.
2 Lacan, J. (1973–1974). *The Seminar of Jacques Lacan Book XXI, the Non-Duped Err.* C. Gallagher (Trans.). Unpublished manuscript, session of 15.1.74.

DOI: 10.4324/9781003712480-15

In losing one language—Sinhala, a language of utility—I didn't simply resort easily to English. Rather, in arriving to an ostensibly English-speaking country—and I say "ostensibly" because the English I encountered when first arriving lacked the grammatical exactitude I had been used to in my few years of schooling prior to arriving—even English, my mother tongue, was rendered strange to me. Such strangeness is something to be taken as of inestimable value. It is what I would many years later take up and endeavour to cultivate as that strange, at times joyful, experience of speaking in analysis.

Many years later again, my relationship to Sinhala began to change. In no longer being a useful speech, it had become fruitful. In occasionally returning now to the country of my birth, I still have no useful facility with the language. Indeed, I cannot really understand a word that is said nor speak a word that could be understood, and yet I enjoy it; the sounds, the lovely musicality of a language which, in not being functional, begins to carry a slice of the fruit of enjoyment.

So, why speak? To cultivate the strangeness of one's own language, the language one claims to be one's own. Such is the domain of a knowledge which is strange in not being the product of a knowing, indeed, arising through the dispossession of a knowing in order to allow a fruitful loving.

In the Seminar of 1973/74, *The non-duped err*, on 11th June 1974, Lacan proposed a mode of operation of the Word with respect to love and to knowledge in contending that it was necessary to be a dupe in order to be in love with one's unconscious. And that it is the non-duped—those who claim to be in the know—who err; who lose their way with respect to love. This was our "only lot in terms of knowledge"[3] but also that of our love.[4]

What might we make from this strange proposition concerning being in love with one's unconscious, with reference to the relationship between the operation of the Word and an approach to love—this being the domain of analysis? It is this relation between the Word and Love which I will place at the forefront of my investigation of the question "Why Speak?"

The title of my chapter—*A Slice of the Word*—is a reference to a provocation made by Lacan in a press conference he gave in Rome in October 1974. This was some four and a half months after the reference to being in love with one's unconscious.

Lacan mused on that occasion that

> you can imagine that I have a certain amount of experience in this sordid profession known as being an analyst. I learned quite a bit there, and this 'In the beginning was the Word' takes on more weight for me. I will tell you something: if there were no Word—which, it must be said, brings jouissance to all those people who come to see me—why would they come back if it weren't to treat

3 Lacan, J. (1973–1974). *The Seminar of Jacques Lacan Book XXI*, session of 13.11.73.
4 Lacan, J. (1973–1974). *The Seminar of Jacques Lacan Book XXI*, session of 23.4.74.

> themselves to a slice of the Word each time? [. . .] It gives them pleasure, they rejoice in it. Without that, why would I have analysands, why would they come back so regularly for years on end?

You can hear in this Lacan's explicit inquiry into the question of *why speak?* His answer is that we seek out a mode of speaking in analysis which affords us that slice of the Word in which we hope to find pleasure and rejoice.

Important to note here is that the slice of the Word which he invokes is not a well-measured, familiar and useful ration. It is not a slice which belongs to the field of utility, even of therapeutic utility, whereby words simply function as a technical means to an end, reduced to their functional aspect of carrying and being carried by meaning. The functional Word as some kind of mediator which effects a reduction in suffering or the cure of a deficiency does not rate a mention here. Rather, it presents itself as a gratuitously lovely slice which is to be served at the table of enjoyment rather than that of meaning.

Therefore, whilst the Discourse of Rome in 1953 acquired the title *The function and field of speech and language in psychoanalysis*, the 1974 press conference in Rome might well be titled *On the possible dysfunction of speech within the field of language*.

The title it did acquire is *The triumph of religion*, and in respect of this slice of the Word, Lacan was familiar enough with the letters of St John to know that the reference "In the beginning was the Word" insists a bit further with: "and the Word was with God, and the Word was God" (John, 1:1). Further, in John 4:8, we find that: "God is love." In this context, the Word is inseparable from love.

In his Papal Encyclical, *Deus Caritas Est*, given in Rome on 25th December 2005 as the first of his papacy, Benedict XVI, addressing himself to the first letter of John (4:8), writes of love, "not as the result of an ethical choice or a lofty idea, but the encounter with an event (a person), which gives life a new horizon and a decisive direction."[5] On the whole, at this point, and from the perspective of analysis, this appears quite promising.

He goes on, however, to render this love *Caritas*. Even when Benedict does cautiously find a place for *Eros* as a love which he defines—somewhat ironically, given that he draws upon the Greek tradition—as "a love between a man and a woman which is neither planned nor willed, but somehow imposes itself upon human beings," it is only on the condition that it submits to renunciation, purification and healing, familiar enough devices of therapeutic utility.[6]

Under the pen of Benedict, love becomes a charitable and therapeutic love—appropriately sanitised as love of the neighbour, bringing benediction to the Word.

5 Benedict XVI, *Deus Caritas Est*. Papal Encyclical of 25th December 2005. Conference of Catholic Bishops, 2006. http://w2.vatican.va/content/benedict-xvi/en/encyclicals/documents/hf_ben-xvi_enc_20051225_deus-caritas-est.html.

6 Benedict XVI, *Deus Caritas Est*, p. 2.

"God is love," under the form of a Christian imperative, becomes a matter of charitable human acts, and in this, theology easily paves a way to a humanistic psychology.

The intent to differentiate psychoanalysis from both theological and psychological perspectives is clear in Lacan's proposition at the beginning of his *Transference* Seminar some 14 years earlier than the press conference in Rome, when he said that

> In the beginning was the Word. If I evoke this, it is to differentiate it from what I am talking about. [. . .]
>
> The "In the beginning" which is pertinent to analytic experience, is love.[7]

How is this different, however, from what is declared in the Gospel of St John?

When Lacan refers to "In the beginning was love" in his *Transference* Seminar, it is certainly not this love of charity, parity and goodness; neighbourly love. It is not his analysand's supposed good which is his concern, but, he says at this point in his teaching, his *Eros*. "I am not there when all is said and done for his good, but in order that he should love."[8] Love understood at this point as *Eros*.

Whilst the Benedictine *Caritas* brings a tidy benediction, it does not furnish that strange slice of the Word bringing with it the pleasure and enjoyment which Lacan argues gives impetus to our speech.

Does this sort out the question then? *Caritas* or *Agape* for Christianity and *Eros* for analysis. It seems like a very promising union, this between analysis and *Eros*. Will Eros therefore be the love which differentiates psychoanalysis such that analysis will there pledge its troth in the vows of holy matrimony? Before finalising the wedding plans for the marriage of psychoanalysis and its apparently chosen love, the handsome *Eros*, let's ask whether he comes from a good family.

Eros is the son of *Penia* (Poverty or lack) and *Poros* (Plenty or surplus)—hovering between want or lack and wealth or excess. According to Diotima, *Eros* is forever in need because of his mother but forever excessive because of his father.[9] This is the Platonic *Eros* in which are conflated love and desire, so unified and unifying as to not augur well for a marriage with analysis, at least after the Lacanian critique. The marriage to *Eros* condemns psychoanalysis to a love in which it is only possible to love what one desires—as lacking. The profit and excesses of *Poros* are neutralised by the losses and deficiencies of *Penia* in a piece of elegant negative gearing, concealing within an economy of desire as a barrier to enjoyment, that slice of the Word which brings an intensification of pleasure and enjoyment. Served

7 Lacan, Jacques. *Transference. The Seminar of Jacques Lacan (1960–1961)*. C. Gallagher (Trans.). Unpublished manuscript, translated from unedited tapes, session of 16.11.60.

8 Lacan, Jacques. *Transference*.

9 In Plato's *Symposium*, Porus was the personification of resourcefulness. He was seduced by Penia whilst drunk at Aphrodite's birthday. Penia subsequently gave birth to Eros.

at the wedding banquet at the marriage of analysis and *Eros*—another Symposium of sorts—is merely a rationed sliver which barely eases the pangs of hunger rather than a gratuitously generous slice which is not at all addressed to deficiency or lack.

Love embodied as *Eros* participates in this double movement, towards poverty and indigence on the one hand—the love peddled by country parish priests—and affluence on the other—that lived by Cardinals. The slice of the Word we seek is to be found in communion with the affluence of love as it tends towards *jouissance* rather than with the poverty of love which finds resigned comfort in desire.[10]

Let's turn our attention, then, to the love with which one might make one's way in analysis—the love which gives the Word its value—and approach this proposition concerning being in love with one's unconscious.

Matthew Del Nevo, a philosopher at the Catholic Institute of Sydney, in addressing himself to Benedict's Encyclical—*Deus Caritas Est*—draws particular attention to the fact that the subtitle is "*de Christiano amor.*" He notes that this word—*amor*—which appears in the subtitle is not discussed in the body of Benedict's text. Indeed, *Caritas* dislodges *amor* to the point where Del Nevo supposes that "There is something unconscious going on therefore."[11] *Amor* is proposed as an unconscious love which has to be redeemed from its dislocation, its repression if you will, in *Caritas* or neighbourly love.[12]

In the writing of St Francis de Sales (1567–1622), specifically in his *Treatise on the love of God*, also published in English as *The Art of Loving God*, Del Nevo finds an author whom he recognises as the principle theorist of amour.[13,14] In this work, we find the strange proposition that the refinement of love is produced through the pursuit of the question of how to make love with God. Firstly, this question—how to make love with God—is a clear provocation in a field which is steadily colonised in the name of a de-eroticised *Caritas*. Secondly, it immediately puts us in mind of the species of love which Lacan invokes with the equally strange notion of being in love with one's unconscious.

Whilst it forms an important critique of the Christian account of love as particularly expressed in Benedict's Encyclical, and therefore its implications for the

10 In the Islamic tradition, this is perhaps more clearly differentiated. In work of Ibn Arabi, for example, writing in the early 1200s, love appears as marked by this same double movement: towards poverty and indigence on the one hand and affluence on the other. It is insofar as love presents itself as an "exceeding in existence" that the creative act which gives rise to the origin of the world and the Word is possible. Ibn Arabî, "Al-Futûhât al-Makkiyya", cited in: de Vos, Idrîs, "L'Amour universal, un cheminement soufi." Librairie Albouraq, Paris, 2013, p. 30.

11 Del Nevo, Matthew. (2015). God is love: In theory. In: *Australian Pentecostal Studies*, vol. 17, p. 4. http:aps-journal.com/aps/index.php/APS/article/view/9479/9482.

12 Might we draw from this that the approach to love which we are investigating in the proposition concerning being in love with one's unconscious is neither *Caritas* nor *Eros* but *Amore*? In Lacan's discourse of ROMA—the press conference of 1974, if not that of 1953—one can't help but be alerted to *AMOR*, the other side—as it were—of ROMA.

13 St Francis de Sales. (2011). *The Art of Loving God*. Cape Cod: Paraclete Press.

14 Del Nevo, M. (2015). God is love.

Word, there are nonetheless, from the point of view of the Lacanian critique, some problems with Del Nevo's position. What particularly allows *Amor* to resist being sanctified to *Caritas*, in his argument, is what we have just problematised as that willing suitor, *Eros*. "*Caritas/Agape* must incorporate *Eros* if it is to be a *living flame of love.*"[15]

Such a conception of love as *Amor*, accompanied by his wingman *Eros*, explicitly conflated in this instance with desire, evokes from Del Nevo the pun: "What could not be *more* natural? Despite this pun between "more" and "amor," which is presented as capable of delivering more, Del Nevo nonetheless falls back into a naturalised reciprocity due to his reliance upon the duplicity of *Eros*. Where Christianity, in perfecting Platonism, is to be found at this place of the conflation of love and desire embraced by Eros, analysis, Lacan contends, holds itself at the place of love, love which is no longer that of *Eros*.[16]

Let's make a pun of our own here as a means of returning to Lacan's proposition made in the Seminar *The non-duped err* and note that, with respect to *Eros*, it is the non-duped—those who are in the know—who err-os; who lose their way with respect to love. *Eros* as the love of those in the know, is to be distinguished from that species of love created in being in love with one's unconscious, whose strangeness we encounter in being its dupe, dispossessed of our knowing.

The Word which is the companion of this love speaks with a strange fluency, the fluency of a strangeness not born of utility but overflowing with the fact that in not being useful, it becomes fruitful. What is at stake, therefore, is a love which tends not towards desire but rather to an intensification of enjoyment. A love which is *Realised* as a knowledge that is no longer the product of a "knowing" but of a "loving"; a being in love with one's unconscious. It is in being the dupe of a knowing as a being in the know that one makes a knowledge through loving.

The proposition concerning "*being* in love with one's unconscious" is, however, perhaps altogether too encumbered by a metaphysical bias with respect to this "being." Let's be mindful also that it is this Christian love as "Divine love" which sutures love to "being" in the assertion "God is love."

There is something, therefore, which we might yet salvage from St Francis de Sales. You will remember Del Nevo's reference to this work as a treatise on how to make love with God. It may allow us to approach Lacan's proposition a little differently. Let us say that it is a question not so much of a "being" in love as of a making love with one's unconscious or of a loving with one's unconscious.

15 Del Nevo, M. (2015). God is love, p. 16. The *Eros* which Del Nevo invokes is defined, then, in the following manner: "For love (*Agape/Caritas*) which is strained to intensity is called desire (*Eros*)." Once again, when we look to *Eros* as a way out of the problematic of love, we end up by conflating love and desire, rendering love as a compensatory love of charity as a balancing, a counterbalancing, of the excess in it. It is this which will lead Lacan to locate Christian love, in its trajectory of the perfection of Platonism, as situating love at the place of desire.

16 Lacan, J. (1973–1974). *The Seminar of Jacques Lacan Book XXI*, session of 18.12.73.

This brings us onto the plane of an originary experience, of love not as a repetition but as a creation. The word not as agent of meaning to be uncovered but as created, manufactured. Such is what arises when the unconscious is *Realised* as a knowledge which is produced not by a knowing but by a loving which, in not seeking the neighbour, seeks the stranger. We encounter this stranger in inhabiting language not knowingly but strangely. This is why we speak in analysis: to encounter the love of the strangeness of language delivered by a very particular slice of the Word.

Such is the approach to love we find in Nietzsche, with whom I began and with whom I will conclude.

> Do I recommend love of the neighbor to you? I prefer instead to recommend flight from the neighbor and love the farthest! Higher than the love of the neighbor is love of the farthest and the future; higher still than the love of human beings is love of things and ghosts. This ghost that runs before you, my brother, is more beautiful than you; why do you not give it your flesh and bones? But you are afraid and run to your neighbor.[17]

17 Nietzsche, Friedrich. (2006). *Thus Spoke Zarathustra*, p. 44.

Chapter 12

Strange effects

Shubha Gokhale

One year, during the holidays, in the period before my analysis was to resume, I began to write a short story in a language I hadn't written one in before: my mother tongue, Marathi. I hadn't planned to write a story in Marathi; far from it. I had never dreamed of doing such a thing. But, on this occasion, suddenly seized by the necessity to write, I began writing what turned out to be a story in epistolary form. A woman is writing a letter to her lover, to her lover who is dead, who has killed himself and so cannot possibly respond to what she has to say. In the letter, she tells a story about a donkey. A donkey is walking across a valley, dusty, mute, heavy with the bags strapped on to its back. Where does it go?

My writing had strange effects: a sense of something having been opened, freed, of having been able to give voice to a disturbance. A sense of excitement, rejoicing, most of all, surprise: How had this happened? My surprise was both because of my ambivalence about Marathi and because I did not rate my proficiency in the language highly. Apart from schoolwork and letters in Marathi to my aunts, I had only ever written anything in English, the first language I learnt to read and write in and the one I have done almost all my reading in.

The effects of this chance writing gave rise to some questions. How do I understand the unexpected freeing effects of my writing in my mother tongue? What makes a language one's own? What does it mean to claim it? Is calling a language 'mine' a question of identity, of culture, love? Does it make sense to speak of discovering a language that was there all along?

Like most Indians who have had an education, I am multilingual. However, because of family circumstances, I had to formally learn to read and write my own mother tongue after the first six-odd years of life. Fluency in the language did not settle the question of *Is it really my language?* Moreover, this uneasiness extended to English as well. This sense of language as fundamentally 'other' is elaborated by Jacques Derrida in his book *The Monolingualism of the Other; or, The Prosthesis of Origin.* Derrida provocatively says, "I only have one language; it is not mine."[1] Derrida, who grew up

1 Derrida, J. (1998 [1996]). *Monolingualism of the Other; or, the Prosthesis of Origin.* P. Mensah (Trans.). Stanford: Stanford University Press, p. 1.

DOI: 10.4324/9781003712480-16

in Algeria at a time when it was a French colony, suffered the predicament of not being fluent in any other language but French but not wishing to call it his mother tongue.

He describes the effects of the violence of colonisation on language rights but asserts that any attempt to find an originary or natural language prior to the colonisation, even one's mother tongue, is doomed, notwithstanding the painful experience of a dispossession. Whence emerge the startling propositions "*We only ever speak one language*" but also "*We never speak only one language*."[2] Historical contingencies aside, language itself is the coloniser, always of the Other and never able to be appropriated absolutely.

While of interest in themselves, both political history and the politics of language seemed peripheral to my own question. I was more struck by Derrida's choice of form: that Derrida *addresses* his argument to an interlocutor. And that his argument problematises the idea of making a claim to a language so that it cannot be settled by an appeal to mastery/proficiency, purity or a superiority of a 'native' language. Derrida appears to claim that estrangement or strangeness is the 'dwelling' of language. Derrida's view of language is similar to Lacan's idea that language inhabits us, that it is not acquired so much as inscribed.

Does the mother tongue have a different status to other languages? The mother tongue, in common parlance, is understood to be the language one has heard spoken by the mother since early life, maybe even the language heard from gestation. For psychoanalysis, the power of the mother tongue is reflected in Freud's idea of the mother eroticising the body of the baby through her taking up of this strange being and making it familiar, familial. Freud spoke about the erotisation of the baby through being held, looked at, spoken and sung to, through being touched by this *langue maternelle*—vulgar, arousing, disturbing (by virtue of being language). Two ideas rich with creative power: the disturbances that come into play by being touched by the mother's tongue and the idea of the address.

Was there any significance to my writing in my mother tongue in the sense of the particular language spoken by my mother? Were the freeing effects to do with the sounds or meanings of that language, used (although not exclusively) in my childhood? To explore this question, it was necessary to look at some ideas about *lalangue* and the mother tongue.

According to Moustapha Safouan, the preponderant place in the formation of *lalangue* is that of the voice: the invocatory object. This idea is traced by Michael Gerard Plastow in his paper presented at the Freudian School of Melbourne in 2023:

> In his book *Lacaniana*, Safouan notes that *lalangue* refers to a language that is singular for each one, transmitted by the first Other that was their mother. Safouan defines it in the following way:
>
>> "It is *not just a question of the mother tongue*, understood as that which the mother spoke, French, English, et cetera, but rather that of *lalangue* in

2 Derrida, J. (1998 [1996]). *Monolingualism of the Other*, p. 7.

> which the subject was from the beginning immersed, of this mother's singular *lalangue*, with the words that were proper to her, her inventions, her funny ways, and from the beginning a signifying equivocation."[3]

Safouan's definition of *lalangue* is touching, with its emphasis on the mother's inventiveness, her "funny ways" and thus her singularity as formative, something the child is informed by without knowing it. The human baby, for so long dependent on the caregiver, is defenceless against the voice; on the other side is the mother, bound to respond to the call of this utterly strange other, born of her body. In the face of this challenge, she draws on her language, her language of everyday use, to invent a response, making something original, trying to find a freedom in this.

From the beginning, speech invokes the other. What do these efforts conjure? Plastow says:

> Lallation is the babbling of the *infans*, taking part in the joy of jabbering, the delight of lallation. But the babbling of the babe endeavours to reach up to the mother's murmurs, a babble that endeavours to construct the oneness of a Tower of Babel in order to reach and to share the mother's tongue. However, as we know, this tower is doomed to collapse as the subject's language, *lalangue inexorably tears the baby away from the mother* [my emphasis].[4]

Lalangue for Lacan was speech not reducible to meaning but speech as resonating; speech as producing disturbances, excitation, thus distinct from a developmental concept that might propose that the first words of the first language learnt in early childhood would constitute *lalangue*. The notion of the purity of a 'first' language is problematised by the experience of a multilingual environment, as in my experience, and the notion of an originary language is problematised by the logic elaborated by Derrida. What is certain is that *lalangue* gets under the skin, producing effects that remain alive, active. Lalangue continues to disturb but is able to be assuaged by an address, in an analysis or a text, a way of giving it its place that might allow one to take up one's own.

The argument that the object of psychoanalysis is the invocatory object and that it allows us to give things new form is developed by Plastow, who says that freedom for the psychoanalytic subject is to do with inventiveness:

> [Freedom] in psychoanalysis is not a freedom to do whatever one chooses. It is rather a constraint upon the subject to unceasingly endeavour to liberate oneself from the images, signifiers, meanings, and contingent objects in which one is caught, in order to destroy these, so that one can continue to create and invent.[5]

3 Safouan, M. (2005). Cited in Plastow, M. (2024). Why the subject is not free? In: *Papers of the Freudian School of Melbourne*. In press.
4 Plastow, M. (2024). Why the subject is not free?.
5 Plastow, M. (2024). Why the subject is not free?, p. 6.

An approach to a making new of speech through an address and its relationship to the question of claiming a language as one's own appears in David Pereira's chapter, "A Slice of the Word," in which Pereira poses and answers the question, *Why Speak?*[6] He argues that speaking in analysis is aimed at an encounter with the strangeness of language. Pereira links this encounter to an idea of love that would be particular to psychoanalysis—a love of excess, of what does not serve a utilitarian purpose. This reference to the slice of the Word comes from Lacan's seminar, *The Non-Duped Err*. Lacan says:

> I will tell you something: if there were no Word—which, it must be said, brings jouissance to all those people who come to see me—why would they come back if it weren't to treat themselves to a slice of the Word each time? [. . .] It gives them pleasure; they rejoice in it. Without that, why would I have analysands, why would they come back so regularly for years on end?[7]

This slice is not readymade. It is the addressing of the other that is pivotal in producing it. There is a *tearing away*, a slicing, an invocation, in addressing the other through speaking—in analysis or through writing. There inheres a brutality, the brutality of the act, in any possibility of freedom and of 'making' in the field of language, whether it is the cutting of a slice of the Word or the destruction of fixed meanings. Whether this act arises from a love of strangeness or from a hatred that must be mined, both love and hate are entwined in the claim there: the equivocation of *(la) mienne/mi-haine*.[8]

Why was I so surprised that I had written in Marathi? I had resiled from calling it mine, always keeping my distance from it—no doubt because it was ever present, providing an insistent and critical internal commentary. I felt caught in two particular moments of speech, which later entered my piece of fiction. First, an experience of being instructed by my mother to do something, with the instruction being uttered at the exact moment that I had begun the very action, with the effect that I was left caught as to whose imperative I was acting on. Second, an experience of protesting against my mother's sharp-tongued criticism and hearing her retort in Marathi: *Do words make holes in your flesh?!* A response that had a muting effect. While these experiences are historical, I carried them around with me for years, at home in the embrace of this commentary. Perhaps the question for me was: what had kept me from claiming this language as my own?

6 Pereira, D. (2024). A slice of the word. In: *Papers of the Freudian School of Melbourne*. In press.

7 Lacan, J. (1973–1974). *The Seminar of Jacques Lacan Book XXI, the Non-Duped Err.* C. Gallagher (Trans.). Unpublished manuscript, session of 13.11.1973.

8 In French *la mienne* means 'mine'; the coinage *mi-haine* suggests something halfway between hate and love (*mi-haine, mi-amour*). *Mienne* and *mi-haine* are homophones in French.

Lacan briefly comments in *Seminar XI* that "in the field of the unconscious the ears are the only orifice that cannot be closed."[9] However, I had resisted being touched, pierced by what I had heard, for the sake of preserving a unity, a oneness of love. This had its price in anguish. At a moment in my analysis, I said: *I don't want to be touched by my mother's words. How can I become immune to them?* The analyst replied: *You can't. But you can do something with what touches you.*

Through the accident of writing those words on to the page, I think that I was able to let the words in and to write and hear Marathi differently, hear what my tongue had to say. A strange freeing of my mother tongue from my mother's tongue. Now it was mine to make up a piece of fiction with. Not my one and only. But mine for as long as it inhabits me. Why write? In order to disturb language, dislodge it from its familiar place. In order to give voice to the disturbances of language. This goes beyond a therapeutic utility, turning what was special coin into common currency that can circulate and be enjoyed. So perhaps the aversion to Marathi, concealed behind the protestation that I was not proficient enough, couched in a familiar formula: *I could never . . . write creatively in Marathi*, sprang from a belief that this mother tongue was my mother's sole domain to enjoy. I could speak it but never in my own way. The imperative to write—interrupted at the moment of its birth by a criticism, or by an instruction to write—thus rendered dubious. Was it mine? Would the words ever be mine?

The erotisation of the mother tongue gets in past all resistance and leaves effects ripe for translation. Writing in the mother tongue then was not exactly a freedom per se but an inventiveness that could make do with history. Since my analysis was conducted in English, it was necessary for me to invent another form in which to address the other in Marathi, to write a fiction. Happy contingency that the holiday break in my analysis meant that I was moved to address the other through writing the story. My mother's words, *Do words make holes in your flesh?!* although wounding, constitute a strange gift. To receive this gift, it was necessary for me to detour through a language I associated with her and to find and write my own associations. To find that I could address other ears: This mother tongue was not lashed to a relation of two beings alone. This was not so much a case of seeking strangeness but of finding it. Answering the call of an otherness that insists produces a writing that is addressed to others. Was this writing born of love? It was born of history, of being pierced, of the attempt to make oneself heard, of chance encounters. The encounter with my mother tongue broke a spell such that I no longer felt at the mercy of that voice and those words, although they remain, indubitably, historical fact.

What fun is it to remain stubbornly united with words that are over-burdened with meaning, complaining all the while that they do make holes in your flesh; but for love of sweet unity, refusing to admit that you are pierced by them? To stop

9 Lacan, J. (1977). *The Four Fundamental Concepts of Psychoanalysis*. J. A. M. Miller (Ed.), A. Sheridan (Trans.). New York & London: W. W. Norton & Company, p. 195.

trying to be immune to what touches me means giving up a fight—this language is neither all mine nor all my mother's—and allows something to pass into a rejoicing that can be mine. Childishly, I delighted in writing as a way of making holes in paper, piercing, imprinting on it, spilling ink, smudging, crossing out, writing over. The donkey in the story crosses the valley again, making its way on dusty legs, the marks left by heavy bags visible on its back. Soon the donkey has passed from sight. Now a braying is heard, strange sonority, a harshness proper to it.

Chapter 13

Of words; their substance and seductions

David Pereira

"Our practice is a swindle," Lacan asserts in an address given in Brussels in February 1977, on hysteria: "Our practice is a swindle, bluffing to make people blink, dazzling them, with words that are a put-on . . ." And yet, he also tells us that "The unconscious has no body but *from* words."[1]

So the clinic of psychoanalysis—constituted by the self-evident fact that it concerns what one says in an analysis—charts a course between a swindle of dazzling words and those "other" words, let's call them, which give body to the unconscious. What particularly continues to interest me in this is the relationship between the word and a certain physicality, the relationship between word and flesh, flesh which at times condescends to being organised and localised as a body. If I say "condescends to being organised as a body," it is to draw your attention to the problematical nature of a body as an organised entity.

The question posed by what the hysteric brings to psychoanalysis concerns the substance of the words uttered by the analyst and the analysand in this peculiar moment of communion called analysis as an encounter convoked by transference.[2] Words which might "carry blood to the speaker's lips and sky to the listener's brow," as exquisitely penned by the blood poet.[3]

If hysteria offers a counter-weight to this propensity to swindling in analysis, it is to the extent that it, hysteria, reminds us that it's not just any words that give body to the unconscious. Nor is it a matter of just any body, as I propose to particularly argue.

Some words, more than others, have the capacity to really touch us, disorganising what we claim to know of ourselves and our bodies. I was, on Thursday the 26th of August 2021, listening to some words uttered in the presence of a body . . . a dead body. The body of someone of whom it could be said, with all the audacity

1 Lacan, J. (1981). Remarks on hysteria: Intervention of Jacques Lacan in Brussels. In: *Quarto*. J. W. Stone (Trans.), no. 2, p. 1.

2 Whilst I acknowledge that there is more than the matter of words uttered, this is nonetheless my focus on this occasion.

3 García Lorca, F. (1998). *Poet in New York*. G. Simon (Trans.). New York: FSG Books, p. 185.

DOI: 10.4324/9781003712480-17

of such a proposition, that we loved each other.[4] In light of the restrictions in force at the time necessitated by the untimeliness of a death in the midst of a pandemic, there were very few of us actually present in the flesh, as it were. It meant that some of the words spoken arrived through the telephone wires, apparently disembodied. And yet, I for one can attest to the fact that these words impacted directly upon the wiring constitutive of that curious thing called my "nervous system"—my very nervous system—causing me to convulse with grief. It is perhaps noteworthy that I did not experience this in a prior moment of gazing upon the dead body in the casket. Only with the uttering of words, even via the telephone wires, did something disorganise my composure—the composition of my body as an organised entity—and overflow to register at the level of my flesh.

My experience, which I do not claim to be entirely unusual, it being present in the very invitation to free associate—to overflow—in analysis, lends a certain freshness—a word which seems obscenely inappropriate given the context, but nonetheless—lends a certain freshness to the question I had already begun to pursue in preparing this chapter. A question which concerns the difference between the symptomatically organised body and a disorganised body given through the word made flesh. It is this difference between "body" and "flesh" which I am alerting you to as central to my argument. I am not using them interchangeably.

Lacan particularly recognised in the offertory of the hysteric this fleshy aspect of the body, the body disorganised and open to making flesh out of the word. In Baltimore on 21st October 1966, he confided that

> When I first began to teach something about psychoanalysis I lost some of my audience, because I had perceived long before then the simple fact that if you open a book of Freud, and particularly those books which are properly about the unconscious, you can be absolutely sure—it's not a probability but a certitude—to fall on a page where it is not only a question of words—naturally in a book there are always words, many printed words—but words which are the object through which one seeks a way to handle the unconscious. Not even the meaning of words, but words in their flesh, in their material aspect.[5]

On Lacan's invitation, if not incitement, let's open one of these books of Freud and consider the status of the words which we find there, words from the Freudian *Corpus*.[6] Opening the pages of the *Studies on Hysteria*, (1893), we find Freud

4 An audacity I commented on in an earlier paper—"For the Love of Safouan"—referencing Derrida's development of the implications of this "we loved each other" in his text "For the love of Lacan" in Derrida, J. (1998). *Resistances of Psychoanalysis*. P. Kamuf, P.-A. Brault and M. Naas (Trans.). Stanford: Stanford University Press.

5 Lacan, J. (1970). Of structure as an inmixing of otherness prerequisite to any subject whatever. In: *The Structuralist Controversy: The Language of Criticism and the Sciences of Man*. R. Macksey and E. Donato (Eds.). Baltimore: The Johns Hopkins University Press, pp. 186–200.

6 In passing, to note here that we are going to discover precisely the difference between opening a book "of" Freud and a book "on" Freud, claiming to represent the Freudian corpus.

outlining the case of Fraülein Elizabeth von R, a "young lady" who presented with a somewhat classical hysterical symptom, suffering from pains in her legs, causing difficulty in walking.[7]

I will not labour the point of the clinical description of this case. Rather, what I want to particularly draw your attention to is Freud's reference in this case to the phenomenon of "conversion," whereby so-called psychical pain is converted into physical symptomatology. In this, the bodily symptom, says Freud, "joins the conversation," drawing our attention to the relationship between words and the body.[8]

In a first analysis of the hysterical presentation, Freud notes that the symptom, the hysterical symptom, is an embodiment given through "the conversion of psychical excitations into something physical."[9] The body lends itself to the staging or organising of the hysterical symptom through a process of "symbolization," to use Freud's term. Whilst this is the familiar enough story, Freud doesn't stop there. What is truly remarkable about hysteria, sufficiently remarkable to warrant Lacan's further remarks on this subject, is to be found in what follows.

Freud goes on:

> In taking a verbal expression literally and in feeling the "stab in the heart" or the "slap in the face" [. . .] as a real event, the hysteric is not taking liberties with words, but is simply reviving once more the sensations to which verbal expression owes its justification.[10]

To this extent, Freud is unequivocally clear: "[H]ysteria is right in restoring the original meaning of the words in depicting its unusually strong innervations. Indeed, it is perhaps wrong to say that hysteria creates these sensations by symbolization."[11] To be clear about the Freudian position: There is something right about this direction of the hysterising of words, in restoring to them a substance which is otherwise lost in a purely figurative or symbolic view. This "Real Event," in which the hysteric is not simply taking liberties with words but invokes a real presence through her body, invites the analytic endeavour to be something other than finding the words to say it. It warrants the analytic adventure as a passage to a Realisation rather than remaining only as a Symbolisation.

Thus we have arrived to the kernel of the Freudian argument concerning the debt owed by psychoanalysis to "hysteria"—hysteria itself—which Freud was capable of separating from the symptomatic hysteric. Lacan, in his turn, made the

7 Freud, S. (1895d [1893–1895]). Studies on hysteria. SE II: 135–181.
8 Freud, S. (1895d [1893–1895]). Studies on hysteria. SE II, p. 148.
9 Freud, S. (1895d [1893–1895]). Studies on hysteria. SE II, p. 157.
10 Freud, S. (1895d [1893–1895]). Studies on hysteria. SE II, p. 181.
11 Freud, S. (1895d [1893–1895]). Studies on hysteria. SE II, p. 181.

same differentiation between the symptomatic hysteric and hysteria itself in claiming for himself the status of an hysteric without symptoms.

The difference I am drawing attention to, therefore, is that between the *symptomatic* hysteric, in whom the word is symbolically organised and re-presented through a body, and the *Real Presence of hysteria itself*, as a fleshing out of the word from its symbolic refuge, the word made flesh. The latter situates the Freudian corpus concerning hysteria quite close to the *corpus Christi*.

Why so?

It concerns the matter of the real presence of Christ in the Eucharist, a concept probably first introduced by Cyril of Jerusalem in the mid-fourth century, and ratified at the Council of Trent in 1551 with the term "transubstantiation." The terms of the debate in 1551 concerned this very question of the difference between the Real Presence of the body of Christ in the sacrament of communion and the symbolic presence of Christ as merely represented in the communion host. Such, I am arguing, is the very tension at play in regard to the substance of words in analysis, which I am pursuing as a question here, drawing on Freud's Real Event of hysteria and Lacan's Baltimore proposition concerning the flesh of words in their material aspect.

In order, then, to continue to flesh out the Freudian position on hysteria, let me offer you another case of the treatment of a hysteric lurching precariously close to a swindle—this time, however, a successful one—whatever is implied by the complete or successful treatment of hysteria.

> [A] woman [. . .] had suffered from haemorrhages for twelve years; and in spite of long treatment by many doctors, on which she had spent all she had, there had been no improvement. On the contrary, she had grown worse. She had heard what people were saying about Jesus, [for that was the name of her physician] so she came up from behind and touched him; for she said to herself "If I touch even his clothes, I shall be cured." And there and then the source of her haemorrhages dried up and she knew in herself that she was cured of her trouble. At the same time Jesus, aware that power had gone out of him, turned around and asked, "Who touched my clothes?" His disciples said to him, "You see the crowd pressing upon you and yet you ask, 'Who touched me?'." Meanwhile he was looking round to see who had done it. And the woman, trembling with fear when she grasped what had happened to her, came and fell at his feet and told him the whole truth. He said to her, "My daughter, your faith has cured you. Go in peace, free forever from this trouble."

The exegesis of this passage from the gospel of St Mark (5: 24–34), which I favour, is one I owe to Graham Ward, Regius Professor of Divinity at Oxford, and to be found in a work of his from 2005 titled *Christ and Culture*, one of the finest pieces of theological scholarship I have read.[12] What particularly struck me about this

12 Ward, G. (2005). *Christ and Culture*. Oxford: Blackwell Publishing.

passage and Ward's exegesis of it is what presents itself as a considerable overlap with the early Freudian case stories: the intimacy of the encounters and the words uttered. If I refer to them as "stories" it is because this is expressly the way Freud referenced them; to be read as "short stories" which immerse us in the intimacy of a real presence and that therefore, Freud writes, "lack the serious stamp of science."[13,14] Freud very interestingly attributed this to the nature of hysteria itself.

It is this double effect of the intimacy of words and the innervation of flesh, something of which I encountered on the abovementioned Thursday the 26th of August 2021, which beckons our further elaboration. Ward's commentary on this passage makes the following argument:

> Perhaps it is because the physicians try to treat the body as a static thing that they fail to heal the woman; they fail to recognise that the body only lives in transit [. . .] located in a "space of flows."[15]

Why is the touch of Christ's body so powerful in this instance? Because, Ward argues, it is in communion with the deterritorialised body of the hysteric; the body of flows and fluid dynamics; the dis-organised body.[16] In Mark's gospel, touch appears not as a direct or pressured touch, as was utilised by Freud in the early treatment of hysterics, but as an *intimation.* Christ's own positioning in this may be considered hysterical, hemorrhagic; that is to say, situated within various operations of flow.

Most significantly, such a touching is capable of delivering a knowledge—as sudden Realisation—which marks itself as different from ordinary comprehension. It constitutes what Ward refers to as an "embodied knowledge," thereby attracting our attention as concerns hysteria, within a theology of embodiment as definitive of Christology. Touch, as a communion with flesh beyond and beneath the body as known, initiates a transferential knowing which is constituted as a *Real Presence*

13 Freud, S. (1895d [1893–1895]). Studies on hysteria, p. 160.

14 As "stories," they give themselves over to what Gregory of Nysa in his Eleventh Homily on the *Canticum Canticorum* (The song of songs, circa 390) describes as the intimacy of the "perception of presence." Werner, J. and Hermann, L. (Eds.). (1960). *Gregorii Nysseni in Canticum Canticorum.* Leiden: Brill, p. 324.

15 Ward, G. (2005). *Christ and Culture*, p. 64.

16 You will note here the influence upon Ward of the Deleuze and Guattarian corpus in locating Christ's touch, the touch of the Word made flesh. See, for example, Deleuze, G. and Guattari, F. (1987). November 28, 1947: How do you make yourself a body without organs. In *A Thousand Plateaus.* B. Massumi (Trans.). Minneapolis: University of Minnesota Press, p. 149. This is a different order of touch than Freud's initial reliance on touch through the "pressure technique" as referenced, for example, in the case of "Miss Lucy R" in Freud, S. (1895d [1893–1895]). Studies on hysteria, pp. 106–124. In this technique, subsequently abandoned in favour of free-association, Freud would use the pressure of his hand upon the head of his patient in order to overcome a resistance to remembering. Either the exercise of pressure or, at other times, the moment of the release of pressure, was intended to facilitate the flow of associations.

rather than a representational knowledge. "Touch is a reaching beyond the boundaries of oneself to find a place not yet given, a future not yet received. It is a gesture of overflow."[17]

In that moment of touch, touch by the word, the body as symptomatically organised is dis-organised and overflows as flesh and nerve in a moment of Realisation. The organised body, through being touched by the word, convulsively opens itself to becoming the Real Presence of flesh. Ward designates this moment of transubstantiation as a trans-corporeal event. For our purposes, this becomes transcorpoREAL, returning us to Freud's assertion of the Real Event of hysteria, as an hysterisation beyond the specific organisation of the hysterical symptom, therefore inviting the possibility of a new relationship to the body given through the intercession of the word as unconscious.

By way of conclusion, and in order to dispel any notion that I am sacramentalising, or indeed mentalising at all, I will have recourse to the transcorporeality offered us by Antonin Artaud once he has done with the judgement of God and made for himself another body.

> All the conceptual systems I may erect never will match these cries of a man engaged in remaking his life [. . .] There are intellectual cries which proceed from the *delicacy* of the marrow. Which I call the Flesh. I don't separate my thought from my life. With each vibration of my tongue I return over the paths of my thought to my flesh.[18]

Artaud makes for himself a "body of flesh and nerve," releasing the Real fleshy presences which innervate his words.[19]

Is this not the mad adventure of psychoanalysis in taking up the path opened by hysteria?

Returning, finally, to Lacan's remarks on hysteria in 1977, he asks where the hysterics of yesteryear had gone, what had replaced those symptoms of old? He answers his own question with the following: "Would not the psychoanalytic craziness have replaced it?"[20] A craziness which, in making Real presence of the word, "can [. . .] carry blood to the speaker's lips and sky to the listener's brow."

Through fleshing out the word which was otherwise caught in either the seductive swindle of dazzling words or its static and fixed embodiment in the hysterical symptom, with Freud and then Lacan, hysteria becomes psychoanalysis.

17 Ward, G. (2005). *Christ and Culture*, p. 67.
18 Artaud, A. (1965). Situation of the flesh. In: *Artaud Anthology*. J. Hirschman (Ed.). San Francisco: City Lights, p. 58.
19 Deleuze, G. (2005). Hysteria. In: *Francis Bacon: The Logic of Sensation*. D. W. Smith (Trans.). London: Continuum, p. 37.
20 Lacan, J. (1981). Remarks on hysteria, p. 1.

Chapter 14

Beyond the word surface

Reading Beckett's *Comment c'est/How It Is* as real writing

Peter Gunn

Is it a novel? This is one of the questions which usually comes up in relation to *Comment c'est/How It Is*. In his magisterial bi-lingual edition of this work, Édouard Magessa O'Reilly says that there is no doubt that it is a novel.[1] Another question is also raised: Is it readable? This essay seeks to take these questions further by asking: Is it writing?

The advent of *Comment c'est/How It Is*

There is an observation, well-known amongst Beckett scholars, that the creation of *Comment c'est/How It* only occurred after an *impasse*. For almost ten years following the publication, in 1953, of *L'innommable*, the last novel of the so-called *Trilogy*, Beckett had produced no new prose works. *Nouvelles et Textes pour rien* was published in 1955, but the pieces assembled under that title had been written in the early 1950s at the latest.

This account appears to receive confirmation from Beckett himself. In a letter written towards the end of 1958 to his lover, Barbara Bray, he says the following:

> I am in acute crisis about my work . . . and have decided that I not merely can't but won't go on as I have been going more or less ever since the Textes pour Rien and must either get back to nothing again and the bottom of all the hills again like before Molloy or else call it a day.[2]

1 This is a much-revised version of an earlier paper, published, in French, in *La Revue des lettres modernes*, 2024–8, n° 9. Comment c'est/How It Is de Samuel Beckett: "ce monde si peu possible", L. Brown (Ed.). Paris: Classiques Garnier, pp. 177–187. My thanks, once again, to the editor, Llewellyn Brown. Thanks also to Megan Williams, the editor of *Papers of The Freudian School*, for her close reading of earlier drafts of this version. O'Reilly, E. M. (2001). *Samuel Beckett Comment C'est How It Is and/et L'Image: A Critical-Genetic Edition/Une Édition Critico-Génétique*, p. x.

2 Beckett, S. (2014). *The Letters of Samuel Beckett, Volume III, 1957–1965*. G. Craig, M. D. Fehsenfeld, D. Gunn and L. M. Overbeck (Eds.). Cambridge: Cambridge University Press, pp. 183–184.

DOI: 10.4324/9781003712480-18

Clearly, however, Beckett did not call it a day. But nor did he himself take an excursion, in the popular psychological sense of "going round the bend." It was in that same year, 1958, that Beckett began working on *Comment c'est*. This text was published in Paris in 1961.[3] *How It Is*, Beckett's own English translation, was published in London in 1964.[4]

In his Seminar *Angoisse*, Lacan reframes such an excursion in psychoanalytic terms, as a departure into the real:

> What is it that [psychiatrists] call a fugue in subjects who have always more or less been put into the infantile position, who cast themselves into it, if not this stage exit, this vagabond departure into the pure world where the subject sets off in search of something that's been rejected everywhere?[5]

Lacan contrasts such a departure into the pure world, which he refers to as the Real, with the aggravations of "going on," that is, the challenges of continuing to take up one's place in the world:

> [O]n one hand [there is] the world, the place where the real bears down, and on the other hand, the stage of the Other where man as subject has to be constituted, to take up his place as the one who bears speech [*la parole*].[6]

This latter, staged world does provide a cover of sorts, "but only ever in a structure that, as truthful as it sets out to be, has the structure of fiction."[7]

In the letter to Bray, Beckett declares that, as an alternative to calling it a day, he might take a turn, a turn back from narration, and, more specifically, from narrating the excursions, over the hills, of his own creations. Even with *L'innommable*, the final novel of the *Trilogy*, published in 1953, we, as readers, can see that there is already a turn. As Simon Critchley puts it, with *L'innommable*, Beckett's narrating voice no longer has a name.[8]

The writing of *Comment c'est/How It Is*

This brings us to what circumscribes this turn: writing itself, in particular, the writing of *Comment c'est/How It Is*.

3 Beckett, S. (1961). *Comment c'est*. Paris: Les Éditions de Minuit.

4 Beckett, S. (2009 [1964]). *How It Is*. E. M. O'Reilly (Ed.). London: Faber and Faber.

5 Lacan, J. (2014 [1963]). *Anxiety: The Seminar of Jacques Lacan Book X*. J.-A. Miller (Ed.), A. R. Price (Trans.). Cambridge: Polity, p. 116. Translation modified.

6 Lacan, J. (2014 [1963]). *Anxiety*, p. 116.

7 Lacan, J. (2014 [1963]). *Anxiety*, p. 116.

8 Critchley, S. (1998). Who speaks in the work of Samuel Beckett? *Yale French Studies*, no. 93, pp. 127–128.

At one level, *Comment c'est/How It Is* can be read as an account of crawling through endless mud in total darkness. In a letter to Donald McWhinnie at BBC Radio Drama dated April 6, 1960, that is to say, before either *Comment c'est* or *How It Is* was published, Beckett himself attempted to summarise "what it's all about":

> A "man" is lying panting in the mud and dark murmuring his "life" as he hears it obscurely uttered by a voice inside him. This utterance is described throughout the work as the fragmentary recollections of an extraneous voice once heard "quaqua on all sides". In the last pages he is obliged to take the onus of it on himself and of the lamentable things it tells. The noise of his panting fills his ears and it is only when this abates that he can catch and murmur forth a fragment of what is being stated within.[9]

This chapter attempts to go beyond any such predigested encapsulation, even one provided by the author. In doing so, it tries to keep pace not with the Beckett who goes on, endlessly, over the hills, but with the relentless "going on" of the writing itself.

Here, ironically, I can do no better than go back to what Beckett himself was saying in 1937, that is, some twenty years before he began working on *Comment c'est*. In a letter to his German friend Axel Kahn, we have the following:

> It is indeed getting more and more difficult, even pointless, for me to write in formal English. And more and more my language appears to me like a veil which one has to tear apart in order to get to those things (or the nothingness) lying behind it. Grammar and style! To me they seem to have become as irrelevant as a Biedermeier bathing suit or the imperturbability of a gentleman [. . .]. To drill one hole after another into [language] until that which lurks behind, be it something or nothing, starts seeping through—I cannot imagine a higher goal for today's writer.[10]

In a series of interviews which Beckett gave to the critic Lawrence Harvey at around the same time as the publication of *Comment c'est* and *How It Is*, Beckett speaks again of the need to get below the surface. He also refers to the sense of an "authentic weakness of being," as well as the unreality of life, of an "existence by proxy," and of the intuition of "a presence, embryonic, undeveloped, of a self that might have been but never got born, an *être manqué*."[11] In order to encounter this

9 Beckett, S. (2014). *The Letters of Samuel Beckett*, pp. 326–327.

10 Beckett, S. (2009). *The Letters of Samuel Beckett, Volume I, 1929–1940*. G. Craig, M. D. Fehsenfeld, D. Gunn and L. M. Overbeck (Eds.). Cambridge: Cambridge University Press, pp. 326–327.

11 Harvey, L. E. (1970). *Samuel Beckett: Poet and Critic*. Princeton: Princeton University Press, pp. 247–248.

otherwise-than-being, there was, for Beckett, a pressing need to get your ear down so as to hear its "infinitesimal murmur."[12,13]

In the present context, we might be reminded of the infinitesimal and anonymous murmurs heard by the narrator of *Comment c'est/How It Is*. Here are the third and fourth fragments of that work:

> *instants passes vieux songes qui reviennent ou frais comme ceux qui passent ou chose chose toujours et souvenirs je les dis comme je les entends les murmure dans la boue*
>
> *en moi qui furent dehors quand ça cesse de halter bribes d'une voix ancienne en moi pas la mienne*[14]
>
> past moments old dreams back again or fresh like those that pass or things things always and memories I say them as I hear them murmur them in the mud
>
> in me that were without when the panting stops scraps of an ancient voice in me not mine[15]

We can note here the use of the word *bribe*/scrap. Somehow, this ancient voice has been given *materiality*. This materiality is paralleled in the writing, as laid out on the page. It consists of a mosaic of disjointed fragments each of which lacks punctuation. As Édouard Magessa O'Reilly points out in his preface to *How It Is*, "[r]ather than units of meaning, these fragments re-configure the narrative as units of breath."[16]

Preliminary to "reading" *Comment c'est/How It Is*, let us then abstain from the periodisation to which authorial biography is prone. Let us, instead, consider this turn of Beckett from an internal perspective, that is, *in terms of what imposes itself in the writing.*

Reading Beckett with Blanchot

For assistance here, we can look to Maurice Blanchot. *Comment c'est/How It Is* could be said to have submitted itself to Blanchot's proposition, first formulated in 1955 in *L'Espace litteraire* [*The Space of Literature*], that the very act of writing brings a passage, "from the first to the third person, so that what happens to me happens to no one, is anonymous insofar as it concerns me, repeats itself in an infinite dispersal."[17]

12 The reference here is to the book by that name by Emmanuel Levinas. (Levinas, E. (1998). *Otherwise Than Being or Beyond Essence*. A. Lingis (Trans.). Pittsburgh: Duquesne University Press).

13 Harvey, L. E. (1970). *Samuel Beckett*, p. 248.

14 Beckett, S. (1961). *Comment c'est*, p. 9.

15 Beckett, S. (2009 [1964]). *How It Is*, p. 3.

16 O'Reilly, E. M. (2009). Preface. Beckett, S. (2009 [1964]). *How It Is*, p. ix.

17 Blanchot, M. (1989 [1955]). *The Space of Literature*. A. Smock (Trans.). Lincoln: University of Nebraska Press, p. 33.

This third person is now, therefore, nothing or at least no person. As Blanchot puts it later, in 1969, in *L'Entretien infini*:

> [To] write is to pass from "I" to "he", but if "he", when substituted for "I", does not simply designate another me any more than it would designate aesthetic disinterestedness [. . .] what remains to be discovered is what is at stake when writing responds to the demands of this uncharacterizable "he".[18]

Speaking of the act of writing, in the "Note" with which *L'Entretien infini* begins, Blanchot describes a radical order of writing which, being concerned only with itself, is without identity:

> Writing, the exigency of writing: no longer the writing that has always (through a necessity in no way avoidable) been in the service of the speech or thought that is called idealist (that is to say, moralizing), but rather the writing that through its own slowly liberated force (the aleatory force of absence) seems to devote itself solely to itself as something that remains without identity, and little by little brings forth possibilities that are entirely other [. . .].[19]

Blanchot goes on to say that this is writing which is "outside discourse, [and even] outside language." To demonstrate the parameters of this outsideness, he compares this order of writing to "the useless notch or the chance groove marked in stone" made by prehistoric humans. Evoking the Événements of May 1968 in Paris, Blanchot also refers to this writing as a *cry* or *murmur* without words: "the written cry, graffiti on the walls."[20]

Reading Beckett with Lacan and Ponge

Jacques Lacan alludes to an order of writing without, or outside, words on several occasions. In 1972, he was giving a series of talks to psychiatrists at Saint Anne Psychiatric Hospital. He orients his audience to this outsideness by evoking the object which he had come to call, since 1957, *objet a*:

> [*Objet a*] has nothing to do with meaning, nor with reason [*raison*]. The question is very pertinent: it's what reason has to do with [. . .] *réson*. Write *r, é, s, o, n*. Write, do it as a favour for me [. . .] It's a spelling of Francis Ponge who, being a poet and, being what he is, a great poet, is not without requiring us, in this question, to take account of what he tells us. He is not the only one. It's a very

18 Blanchot, M. (1993 [1969]). *The Infinite Conversation*. S. Hanson (Trans.). Minneapolis: University of Minnesota Press, p. 380. For the discussion of Blanchot which follows I am indebted to Kuzma, J. D. (2019). *Maurice Blanchot and Psychoanalysis*. Leiden: Brill Rodopi.

19 Blanchot, M. (1993 [1969]). *The Infinite Conversation*, p. xii.

20 Blanchot, M. (1993 [1969]). *The Infinite Conversation*, p. 262.

grave question that I have only seen seriously formulated, outside this poet, at the level of mathematicians.[21]

In a footnote, there is a quote from Ponge from his collection of essays *Pour un Malherbe*, as follows: "*raisons, résons: un concert de vocables, de sons significants* [reasons, *résons*: a concert of terms, of significant sounds]."[22,23]

Quoting from the same collection, the French critic Michel Collot summarises Ponge's position as follows:

> If the poet does not limit himself to reproducing "objects of the external world", but transforms them into objects of art, it is because he imprints and "expresses" his inner complexes upon them. The materiality of the signifier and the thickness of meaning are also "material for expression", a "reserve of sentimental impulses". If their "play" can assume a certain "interest", and even a real "gravity", it is because a subject brings into play what is most intimate to him:
>
> *It is a matter of expressing something; and what? something differential, something particular*, the most particular sensitivity, *the heartstring* [*la corde sensible*].[24]

This recalls what Lacan says to the psychiatrists: "In other words [. . .] reason (of which we will limit ourselves to saying that it starts from the grammatical apparatus) has to do with something that would impose itself [. . . it has to do] with something *resonant*."[25]

As I read Lacan reading Ponge, in certain circumstances, certain intimate circumstances, such differential resonances can become intrusive, even traumatic. Yet, wonders Lacan, might it be the case that reason, and indeed reality itself, is made from such heart-breaking impositions?

> Is what resonates, the origin of the *res* ["thing" in Latin], what "reality" is made from? It's a question, a question that touches very properly speaking, on all that can be excerpted from language, in the name, in the name of logic [. . .]. And it is there that the question is posed of where the real is centred from [. . .]. There are mathematicians who say that [. . .] there is something beyond [. . .] which seeks beyond to that which *réson* (*r,é,s,o,n*) takes recourse regarding what is in question, in other words some Real.[26]

21 Lacan, J. (2013 [1972]). *The Knowledge of the Analyst/Le savoir du psychanalyste: The Seminar of Jacques Lacan 1971–1972*. M. Plastow (Ed.). Paris: l'Association Lacanienne internationale, pp. 99–101. Translation modified. For more on *objet a*, I refer readers to Allouch, J. (1998). How Lacan invented *Objet a*. In *Papers of the Freudian School of Melbourne*, vol. 19, D. Pereira (Ed.), P. Anderson (Trans.). Melbourne: The Freudian School of Melbourne, pp. 1–3.

22 In French, '*résonner*' means "to resonate."

23 In French, '*résonner*' means "to resonate," p. 101, n. 9.

24 Collot, M. (1993). *Entre mots et choses*. Seyssell: Champ Vallon, p. 184. My translation.

25 Lacan, J. (2013 [1972]). *The Knowledge of the Analyst/Le savoir du psychanalyste*, p. 101.

26 Lacan, J. (2013 [1972]). *The Knowledge of the Analyst/Le savoir du psychanalyste*, p. 101. Translation modified.

Lacan goes on to make use of a short poem by Antoine Tudal. The poem's opening lines are as follows,

> *Entre l'homme et la femme,*
> *Il y a l'amour*
>
> [Between man and woman,
> There is love]

For Lacan, what distinguishes these lines from doggerel is that, in speaking them, something else can be heard, beyond the words; a *hum,* a *resonance.* This "something that would impose itself" comes from between, in this case, from the lacuna between man and woman.

> "Between man and woman, there is love", that means that . . . [Lacan strikes his hands] Eh! It sticks—a world, it floats. But with: "There is a wall", there, you understand that "*between*" means "interposition."[27]

As I read Lacan here, inspired by the poet, and hearing his own saying of this very poem *resonating* from the walls of the auditorium at Saint Anne, he comes to *Real*-ise, with a jolt, that he himself is, in that moment, excerpted from this *scenario.* It is for this reason/*réson* that for Lacan, the outside, otherwise known as the between, is *love.*

Reading *Comment c'est/How It Is* with *Foirades/Fizzles*

If *Comment c'est/How It Is* is writing which seeks to touch on such extremity, how might we read it?

To start with, this must be a reading where the unit of attention extends beyond any sequence of words, however coherent they might appear in isolation, to encompass the textual fragment within which that sequence lies and, beyond that, to the very *fabric of the page.*

In summary, this must be a *material* reading, one which is more concerned with the *materiality* of the text as it presents itself to us *in the act of reading* than it is with words in their supposedly sovereign meaning.[28] Such a reading pays attention

27 Lacan, J. (2013 [1972]). *The Knowledge of the Analyst/Le savoir du psychanalyste*, p. 107.

28 Many critics have pointed out that Beckett's work undercuts any attempt to give words fixed meaning. This has the effect of generating new ways of reading. Quoting what Beckett said in 1930 in *Proust,* Carla Locatelli notes that Beckett, in privileging the practice of art over that of interpretation, gives a limit to this multiplication:

> Beckett's works remain "hieroglyphics", not only because time proves that many new possibilities of reading develop around and because of them, but also because the resistance to a final semantic appropriation of their meaning compels interpretations to multiply, ever to be engulfed by "an art that is perfectly intelligible and perfectly inexplicable."

to the white space between and around the fragments, that is, to what lies *outside* the fragments considered as text. From another point of view, this is a reading which encompasses the nothing which lies in between.

Such a reading is fostered by having the French and the English versions of *Comment c'est/How It Is* side by side. This is what Edouard Magessa O'Reilly's critical-genetic edition enables.[29] We see then that in order to align the text of the various small fragments which, at one level, can be read as comprising the text of each version, the amount of white space must vary. Ironically, this attempt to correlate the two versions only draws attention to what lies beyond them both: nothing.

Some further indication of the orientation which this order of reading requires is given by *Foirades/Fizzles*. I am referring to the artists' book by that title. This was published in a limited edition in 1976, that is, fifteen years after *Comment c'est.* Here, thirty-three non-representational etchings by Jasper Johns are intercalated with five previously unpublished texts by Beckett, which he called *foirades* or, in English, "fizzles".[30]

This work was not a collaboration in the usual sense. Johns designed the book, aided by Mark Lancaster, his assistant. Beckett allowed Johns to determine the way in which the *foirades/fizzles* were arranged, and it was Johns's decision to present them in both their French and English versions. Johns chose five of the *foirades*, which Beckett then translated into English. Johns's etchings were based on an existing work, *Untitled*, a four-panel painting from 1972.[31]

Despite the lack of formal collaboration, some degree of "cohabitation" can nevertheless be discerned. But this presents itself not at the level of the individual but *at the level of the fabric of the work itself.* For that reason, it manifests itself in the *act*, the act of reading, and also, and in conjunction with that, the act of making, of fabrication.

Locatelli, C. (1990). *Unwording the Word: Samuel Beckett's Prose Works after the Noel Prose.* Philadelphia: University of Pennsylvania Press, p. 3.

29 O'Reilly, E. M. (Ed.). (2016). *Samuel Beckett Comment c'est How It Is and/et L'image, a Critical-Genetic Edition Une edition critic-génétique.* New York: Routledge.

30 According to Marjorie Perloff:

> Fizzles (farts, hissing sounds, failures) is a mild translation of *Foirades* which means "shit" or "diarrhea." The Jasper Johns–Samuel Beckett collaboration *Foirades/Fizzles* was published in a limited signed edition of 250 copies by Petersburg Press, South America, 1976. The etchings were proofed and printed at the Atelier Crommelynck in Paris in 1975–1976. The publication was edited by Vera Lindsay, who conceived of the project and brought Beckett and Johns together. (Perloff, M. (1983). 'The space of a door': Beckett and the poetry of absence. In: *The Poetics of Indeterminacy, Rimbaud to Cage.* Evanston: Northwestern University Press, p. 201).

The six texts, together with two new ones, were published separately, in both the original French and in Beckett's own English translation, as follows: Beckett, S. (1976). *Pour finir encore et autres foirades.* Paris: Minuit; and Beckett, S. (1976). *Fizzles.* New York: Grove Press. See also Nixon, M. (2010). *Preface to Texts for Nothing and Other Shorter Prose, 1950–1976.* London: Faber, pp. xvii–xviii.

31 Goldman, J. (1977). Introduction. In: *Foirades/Fizzles.* New York: Whitney Museum of American Art.

In a brilliant essay, the art historian Richard S. Field shows us how Johns, in company with Beckett, demonstrates this. He takes the example of *Words (Buttock Knee Sock . . .)*.[32]

Field sees this pair of etchings as emblematic of the whole project. It is placed towards the beginning of the book, between the French and English versions of the first of Beckett's *foirades*. It is preceded by two etchings, the first of which appears to show the numeral "1" in large Roman lettering, but with the upper right-half of the image-space covered in scribbles. This is despite the fact that, in the separate published versions of the texts of the *foirades/fizzles*, this one is listed fourth. The second etching appears to be a mistake. It shows what looks like a smudge of watery ink, with drips coming from the left-hand corner, and with a large black "X" towards the lower right side.

At one level, the etching *Words (Buttock Knee Sock . . .)* consists of two lists, in bold type, of words associated with the body: buttocks, knee, sock, foot, hand, floor, face, torso, leg, feet. The list on the left is in English, the one on the right is in French. In the case of both lists, however, these "body-words" are printed over the corresponding words in French or English, respectively. Furthermore, these "shadow" words are in reverse letter order and in type which appears faded.

Having gone into some detail about the complexities of Johns's production process for *Words (Buttock Knees Sock . . .)*, Field makes a brilliant observation:

> Johns had mimicked the process of translation in a way that suggested a lingering presence of the original language. And he equated that act of translation with the specific action of reading this book of French and English texts. What is more, the words themselves suggest an even greater mystery of language, namely its ability to substitute a sign, a word, a name, for an object. Johns even manages to infiltrate the subtler question, of how one thing, buttocks for example, can be represented by both the English and the French words; are they the same? This question of identity pervades the whole of Johns' work, and especially the images and texts of *Foirades/Fizzles*.[33]

This particular etching also manages to infiltrate an even more fundamental question of identity. Keeping to the fabric of the page, this is identity not at the level of the individual but at the level of *writing*. Furthermore, although it must pay its respects to language, this is writing which makes its presence felt by what it demonstrably excerpts from language: the act of making no more than a mark.

32 Field, R. S. (1988). The making of Foirades/Fizzles. In: *Foirades/Fizzles: Echo and Allusion in the Art of Jasper Johns*. J. Cuno (Ed.). Los Angeles: Grunwald Center for The Graphic Arts, pp. 103–104.

33 Field, R. S. (1988). The making of Foirades/Fizzles, pp. 103–104.

Reading *Comment c'est/How It Is* with love

What does this tell us about reading *Comment c'est/How It Is* at this level?

We might do well, first of all, to recall Leslie Hill's observation that "Written and murmured across the excrement [. . .] the words of *Comment c'est* exist as so many marks, traces, stains, smudges and inscriptions spelt out over the page, letter by letter."[34] He goes on to refer to that excrement as "the remains of what has been expelled from a body in its attempt to sign its place in language."

With the Beckett of *Comment c'est/How It Is* and *Foirades/Fizzles*, however, the reader is held not by the narrative, such as it is, but by *the shit*; that is, not by the words but by *the remains of the words*. It might be better therefore to say that this excrement only signs a place inasmuch as it can be read as beckoning to a place beyond, or, even better, between the word surface.

Such a reading holds considerable danger, as Blanchot tells us. If the reader finds herself called by this siren without words, that resonance might be so great that she too risks "going round the bend." But, finding herself caught up in that roundabout, that *étourdit*, she might also, for that very *réson*, *fall*, fall in love.[35] From that place, that fallen place of love, new possibilities might arise.

34 Hill, L. (1990). *Beckett's Fiction, in Different Words*. Cambridge: Cambridge University Press, p. 139.

35 *L'étourdit* is a text by Lacan. The title draws in part on that of Moliere's comedy of errors, *L'étourdi*. It can be translated in numerous ways, including "the scatter-brained one," "the amazed said" or "the dizzy turn." More importantly however, as Christian Fierens tells us in his *A second reading of Lacan's Etourdit*, *l'étourdit* turns around the turn (*tour*) and the said (*dit*) where meaning lapses into absurdity (*l'étourderie*).' (Fierens, C. (2014). *A Second Reading of Lacan's Etourdit*. C. Gallagher (Trans.). http://www.lacaninireland.com/web/wp-content/uploads/2010/06/Fierens-2nd-reading-of-etourdit-May-2014.pdf, consulted May 2025. Translation modified). Fierens goes on:

> "Tu ne sauras jamais combien je t'ai aimé." [You will never know how much I loved you] Addressed to a woman, that may stir things up, but that is not what is important. The forgotten "e" [in the session of December 19, 1972 of his Seminar *Encore*, Lacan mentions having made a slip of the pen; in a letter addressed to a woman he wrote *aimé* instead of *aimée*], the silent "e" begins to speak of itself and it is love which speaks itself and of itself, the love letter, without appealing to the documentation of some diagnostic or police-style suspicion. A single letter. *L'étourdit* offers us its silent "t". It is enough to make *l'étourdi* and the unconscious speak.

Chapter 15

Beyond the pale

Megan Williams

> Lacan on woman:
>
> A woman can but be excluded by the nature of things, which is the nature of words.[1]
>
> Woman cannot be said.[2]
>
> She is called woman (*dit femme*) and defamed (*défame*).[3]
>
> There is a jouissance [. . .] a jouissance of the body [. . .] 'beyond the phallus'.[4]
>
> Lacan on man:
>
> He animates nothing—he takes the other as his soul.[5]
>
> [W]hen one is a man, one sees in one's partner what one props oneself up on [. . .] narcissistically.[6]

In the novel *Milkman* by Anna Burns, woman is called "cat".[7] Cats are murdered by men and boys. Cats are:

> vermin, subversive, witch-like, the left hand, bad luck, feminine, [. . .] not adoring like dogs. They don't care. They can never be relied upon to shore up a human ego. They go their way, do their thing, are not subservient.[8]

1 Lacan, J. (1998). *The Seminar of Jacques Lacan, on Feminine Sexuality: The Limits of Love and Knowledge: Book XX. Encore 1972–1973*. B. Fink. (Trans.). New York & London: W. W. Norton & Company, p. 73.
2 Lacan, J. (1998). *The Seminar of Jacques Lacan, on Feminine Sexuality*, p. 81.
3 Lacan, J. (1998). *The Seminar of Jacques Lacan, on Feminine Sexuality*, p. 85.
4 Lacan, J. (1998). *The Seminar of Jacques Lacan, on Feminine Sexuality*, p. 74.
5 Lacan, J. (1998). *The Seminar of Jacques Lacan, on Feminine Sexuality*, p. 82.
6 Lacan, J. (1998). *The Seminar of Jacques Lacan, on Feminine Sexuality*, p. 87.
7 Burns, A. (2018). *Milkman*. London: Faber and Faber Ltd.
8 Burns, A. (2018). *Milkman*, p. 93.

DOI: 10.4324/9781003712480-19

A man cannot take a cat as his soul.

I have called my Chapter "Beyond the pale". Urban Dictionary tells us that the phrase:

> dates back to the 14th century, when the part of Ireland that was under English rule was delineated by a boundary made of stakes [. . .] and known as the English Pale. To travel outside of that boundary, *beyond the pale*, was to leave behind all the rules and institutions of English society, which the English modestly considered synonymous with civilization itself.[9]

Wikipedia confirms this meaning and adds: "Also derived from the 'boundary' concept was the idea of a pale as an area within which [only] local laws were valid".[10] Wiktionary comments that the boundary of Ashdown Forest (a royal hunting forest) was also known as the Pale, consisting of a paled fence and a ditch inside, to allow deer to jump in but not back out.[11]

The phrase resounds throughout *Milkman*. Although the novel is set in what one assumes is a city in Northern Ireland, the order of civilisation within the pale here is made not by the English but by the "renouncers-of-the-state", those who fight with weapons of terror against that colonising country "over-the-water". Nevertheless, the two adversaries are mirror images of each other—the fight is conducted in repetitive, complementary, almost choreographed encounters between renouncers and enemy forces, each ruled by the same discourse of mastery which includes the orienting of sexual difference according to the phallic order. It is not the enemy which is beyond the pale, then, but the subversive, feminine beings who transgress this order by displaying an other enjoyment, a "jouissance beyond the phallus."[12] They do not form a category which could constitute an adversary and cannot be regarded as making exceptions to the All-Within-the-Pale set, since they are multiple and potentially infinite in their variation.

Beyond the pale, for instance, is the sunset brought to the attention of the class by the French teacher, and thus the French teacher herself, and even the practice of attending French class. *Look!* the teacher says to the class (I am paraphrasing her), *Look at the sunset and all the colours that burst forth from it: green, pink, blue, yellow, violet, indigo. See them shift and change, feel the movement, breathe it in, be inspired, be excited. Take up this sunset as a sensual practice rather than a concept.*[13] *Non*, the French class replies, *le ciel est bleue! Le ciel est bleue!*, and

9 https://www.urbandictionary.com.
10 https://en.wikipedia.org/wiki/The_Pale.
11 https://en.wiktionary.org/wiki/beyond_the_pale.
12 Lacan, J. (1998). *The Seminar of Jacques Lacan, on Feminine Sexuality*, p. 103.
13 Deleuze and Guattari argue for a practice which cultivates the sensual in order to resist the congealing effects of the conceptual. Deleuze, G. and Guattari, F. (2013). *A Thousand Plateaus*. London & New York: Bloomsbury Academic, pp. 134–150.

What's the point? There's no point! in looking at a sunset.[14] What the teacher says has no symbolic value in their order. *And* the teacher is a woman.

Also beyond the pale, although the community doesn't yet know it, is maybe boyfriend of the heroine, maybe boyfriend who is maybe hetero, maybe hommo, certainly the lover of chef, who *is* hommo; lover as well of those well-known hommo fascinations of cooking and coffee pots, sunsets and *petits fours* and other unmanly, pointless things.[15] They are becoming just like women.[16]

Again beyond the pale is the real milkman, also known as the man who doesn't love anybody. Note the singular. Real milkman doesn't love any *single* body, single object determined by history, Oedipus, fantasm, loss, but instead loves everybody—in the sense of accepting everybody's transference. When the woman he loved loved God more than him, he found that he could not replace her and make a series. Rather than repeat the same trajectory of desire caused by lack *encore*, he founds a new practice each time he travels, transiting the surface in his milk van, loving all the women, open to all occurrences, listening to all speech, washed through by intensities that surge and pass, each time different. Perhaps he is becoming-woman.

Also beyond the pale is the heroine of the novel. She is the girl who walks, who goes her own way, does her own thing: does it in public by walking-while-reading or reading-while-walking, the words separated by hyphens, indicating a continuing, something which does not build towards a point and then crest and discharge only to begin again but rather continues, transiting, wandering, meandering across the surface without aim or end point. She walks-while-reading everywhere, day and night, evoking the words of Cixous and Clément: "She goes on and on infinitely [. . .] able not to return to herself [. . .] her rising not an erection but a diffusion."[17] Walking-while-reading 19th-century novels, she is vigilant in her refusal of the vigilance towards her own century which renouncer law demands of

14 Burns, A. (2018). *Milkman*, pp. 69, 70.

15 The double "m" refers to Lacan's usage of the word *hommosexuel*, intended to emphasise the man, *homme*. In Lacan's view, loving a man is always *hommosexuel*, whether the lover is a man or a woman, since it is the phallic sexual orientation that forms a set within which all are the same in being subject to castration, or sexual desire arising from lack. The hetero, or other, falls on the side of women, since they do not form a set; they are not all the same in their jouissance and have to be taken one by one. Thus he argues that Woman does not exist. Lacan, J. (1998). *The Seminar of Jacques Lacan, on Feminine Sexuality*, p. 85.

16 Félix Guattari argues that all becoming—and becoming is given a value above and beyond identity—transitions first through becoming-woman. The reason for this is that woman is still close to, indeed, participating in, the phallic order. Therefore, to become beyond the phallic order—to become animal or vegetable—one must first become woman. Guattari, F. (1984). Becoming a woman. In: *Molecular Revolution: Psychiatry and Politics*. London: Peregrine Paperbacks, pp. 233–235. Thanks to David Pereira for his introduction to and commentary on this work in his seminar, Psychoanalysis, Philosophy and Theology.

17 Cixous, H. and Clément, C. (1986). *The Newly Born Woman*. Minneapolis: University of Minnesota Press, p. 88.

the community, disorienting herself from its orientation, enacting a sexuality that has "zero symbolic value".[18] In a community ordered by a history that will not stop not stopping, that never ceases to repeat its cyclical discharge of tension, she seems to embody the excessive, surplus presence of erotic tensions which history cannot discharge because that jouissance is not organised by its sameness to something lost—each time she walks, there is no point, no loss, no nostalgia and no repetition. Going her own way, doing her own thing, she is a cat, a fact pointed out by Somebody McSomebody, her stalker, when he corners her in the toilets of a nightclub. Going her own way, doing her own thing, she draws to her the masculine McSomebodies of the pale, compelled—by the outrage of a beyond—to possess, colonise, organ-ise a jouissance that has no point . . . of discharge, because it is without the organ that focuses masculine narcissism. Most potently of all, going her own way draws to her the milkman, to make her go his way.

Real milkman is "real" insofar as he is not *the* milkman, who is not a milkman. The milkman is the lethal, eponymous, overshadowing presence of the novel, "Man of Men, Warrior of Warriors, our high-celebrity, local community hero".[19] He is the power, the bomber, the predator. The milkman *is* the phallic All, *is* the pale, is the focused point of All the men fighting the binary other to a discharge of jouissance *encore*: for the men, there is a point.[20] They still have something to lose—*encore*.[21]

So the milkman is drawn to the girl who walks, to subjugate the beyond of his power, to make a hole in the surface, to become the cause that penetrates her jouissance. She begins to find him beside her, come apparently from nowhere or from everywhere, running with her when she runs, offering the open door of a car when she reads-while-walking, speaking quietly as though in the continuation of a conversation which they have always been having, as though they are a couple, looking straight ahead and naming her family, friends, place of work and maybe-boyfriend, the latter embedded in a roundabout, indirect discourse about car bombs which could only be a threat except that no threat is spoken. He never threatens, only once looks at her, never touches her, simply acts as though it's certain that they, the two of them, are heading ineluctably towards an end point which is already written or maybe already arrived at, which both of them know. His discourse surrounds and confuses her, and she is slowly herded towards his goal, aided in this by the entire community, which assembles to gather her in, make her jump inside the pale: her family and the sanctities (praying women) by assuming she is already his and lecturing her about being the mistress of a paramilitary; the girlfriends of the other

18 Cixous, H. and Clément, C. (1986). *The Newly Born Woman*, p. 42.

19 Burns, A. (2018). *Milkman*, p. 176.

20 Lacan's formulation of sexual difference, referred to in *fn* 2, regards masculine sexuality as making a set within which All men are located, unlike feminine sexuality, which cannot be so defined as to make a set of women. Lacan, J. (1998). *The Seminar of Jacques Lacan, on Feminine Sexuality*.

21 On this point of having something to lose, see Cixous, H. and Clément, C. (1986). *The Newly Born Woman*, p. 87.

paramilitaries by closing around her in the toilets of a nightclub and regaling her with lipstick, perfume and advice about how to live with the risk, excitement and power of being a girlfriend of the secret controllers, the bombers, the hunted, the state which is the lining of the official state; the status quo.

His pursuit and their herding wear her down. She begins to falter, forget, ask herself "What's the point? There's no point".[22] Relations deteriorate: with her mother due to lectures on ordinary, womanly duties versus the infernal excitement of paramilitaries; with work due to her repeatedly interrupting sleep to make sure that the milkman hasn't gotten into her room at night; with the community due to her stubborn presentation of a blank, inert face to its gossip, which leads, contrary to her intention, to a dispossession of herself:

> [M]y feelings stopped expressing. Then they stopped existing. And now this numbance from nowhere had come so far on in its development that along with others in the area finding me inaccessible, I, too, came to find me inaccessible. *My inner world, it seemed, had gone away*.[23]
>
> . . . Even the walking was coming to a halt [. . .] a lameness of stance setting in and overtaking me.[24]

She withdraws from maybe-boyfriend to keep him safe from the milkman and then also because she begins to be repulsed by him, his touch somehow evoking that of the milkman even though this was incomprehensible because the milkman had never touched her. And similarly, because nothing physical has happened, which means nothing *has* happened, she can't ask for help—along with everyone else, she holds the belief:

> about someone not doing something so how could they be doing it—which meant how could I open my mouth and threaten widespread disintegration of the current status quo?[25]

Cixous and Clément:

> They have committed an anti-narcissism on her! A narcissism that only loves itself if it makes itself loved for what is lacking.[26]
>
> They are going to help her become a subject [. . .] by making her guilty.[27]
>
> She must resist just long enough for him to feel his power and desire and give him the pleasure of enjoying the return to himself.[28]

22 Burns, A. (2018). *Milkman*, p. 185.
23 Burns, A. (2018). *Milkman*, p. 178.
24 Burns, A. (2018). *Milkman*, p. 185.
25 Burns, A. (2018). *Milkman*, p. 64.
26 Cixous, H. and Clément, C. (1986). *The Newly Born Woman*, p. 68.
27 Cixous, H. and Clément, C. (1986). *The Newly Born Woman*, p. 46.
28 Cixous, H. and Clément, C. (1986). *The Newly Born Woman*, pp. 79–80.

When she has resisted enough, when "everything has microscoped down to that one last threshold" of getting into his car and she can no longer find the point of refusal, he knows it.[29] He pulls up in his car, opens the door, and she jumps in to the pale, to impalement. She describes the moment that the milkman's fantasy reaches its culmination:

> [H]e turned [. . .] in his seat towards me. Finally I felt the gaze, the long, slow gaze, upon me, because now he could [. . .] allow himself to look. Here was success, completion, property. In contrast, I was the one who remained this time looking ahead.[30]

They have made the deer jump in. He will take her as his soul. He voices the scene of his fantasy to her: At night, he will call for her in one of his cars, and she will come out to him and not keep him waiting, wearing: "Not trousers. Something lovely. Some feminine, womanly, elegant, nice dress".[31] He will come every night until another deer wanders past, ignoring him, and he has to chase it down.

An analysand in my clinic speaks of a rape in her childhood. She says that a darkness without limit opened at the moment of experiencing that the words that she spoke to this familiar man had no effect on his act. The threshold of womanhood: *Her words had no effect.* In the unlimitedness of that dark, she became a creator: She operated a grammatical negation that removed her from his act and extended her self into another space, another time, in which she left his act behind, was ignorant of him, wandered off and did not return to that self; transitioned; became a woman. This is what makes men kill women: that women can leave them, wandering elsewhere.

It is what made the men of the novel want to kill *real* milkman: his wandering, transiting and ignoring of their manly pursuits. He wasn't interested in their exploits; threw the guns they had buried in his cellar out into the street, for which they planned to kill him.

When the men captured him and took him into a hut to execute him, they suddenly found their hut surrounded by all the women of the district, silently sitting and pointing, making an accusing shape that could be seen from above by any helicopter of the state that happened to be surveilling. The men were astonished—and checkmated. These women were their loyal protectors, their own wives and mothers, the homespun medical corps who billeted renouncers, tipped them off about informers, transported weapons, sounded alarms at the approach of the state, sewed up wounds and dispensed homemade remedies—but here, they crossed a pale that the men had thought immutable. There aren't two Gods, says Lacan, but

29 Burns, A. (2018). *Milkman*, p. 136.
30 Burns, A. (2018). *Milkman*, p. 299.
31 Burns, A. (2018). *Milkman*, p. 300.

there isn't just one either—God has a woman face and so do these women.[32] The event seized them, and they acted. With one face turned to philía, the soullove of masculine discourse, but another, perhaps for the first time, turned away from the men, they demanded relentlessly, obstinately, immovably of these husbands and sons, now enemy, that their friend the real milkman was to be released "fully intact and breathing"[33].[34] The men have until now taken these becoming-women as use value only. Now they are commanded by this instant eruption of passion and creativity.

David Pereira's Melbourne seminar Psychoanalysis, Philosophy and Theology introduced an extensive reading and commentary on various works of Gilles Deleuze and Felix Guattari, including "Becoming a Woman." Reading the latter, I wondered why Guattari regards feminine becoming as the starting point for any becoming.[35] His answer to this question, and the novel *Milkman*'s, can perhaps be rendered in Lacan's terminology. It's because God has two faces; because there is no one which is not phallic and yet some are not-all so.[36] A woman—which anyone can choose, Lacan says—is in discourse as well as being open to a jouissance beyond it; not phallically organ-ised. She is subject to philía, to hommosexuality, as well as open to sexual otherness. This un-sayable of a woman transitions beyond the wall of language, not by *being* something else—which could be said—but by necessity *as* a *becoming*—a becoming-woman which may then lead to other forms of becoming.[37]

Real milkman, *à l'envers* the discourse of the master, is the milkman's double, his becoming-woman, his feminine shadow thrown wandering beyond the pale, where the truth of power falls onto the real.[38] Real milkman demonstrates how the discourse of psychoanalysis walks-while-listening in and out of the real: He receives and witnesses that jouissance which is trans, unrepresented, without a place. The girl-who-walks, one night after French teacher disturbs her into actually seeing, for the first time ever, the colour in a sunset, comes, in an interstitial space,

32 Lacan, J. (1998). *The Seminar of Jacques Lacan, on Feminine Sexuality*, p. 77.

33 Lacan makes a play on the homophony in French of the first syllable (*ame*) of love (*amour*) with the word for soul (*âme*). His argument is that hommosexual love is one in which "the soul souloves the soul (*l'âme âme l'âme*) [and thus] sex is not involved," since sex involves otherness, rather than taking the other for one's soul. Lacan, J. (1998). *The Seminar of Jacques Lacan, on Feminine Sexuality*, p. 84.

34 Burns, A. (2018). *Milkman*, p. 322.

35 Guattari, F. (1984). Becoming a woman, pp. 233–235.

36 Lacan, J. (1998). *The Seminar of Jacques Lacan, on Feminine Sexuality*, pp. 72–80.

37 Lacan used the term "the wall of language" in 1953 in reference to the following poem by Antoine Tudal (2000). Between man and love, / There is Woman. / Between man and woman, / There is a world. / Between man and the world, / There is a wall. Lacan, J. (2002). *Ecrits: The First Complete Edition in English*. B. Fink (Trans.). New York: W. W. Norton & Company, pp. 233, 239.

38 Lacan designated the discourse of analysis as *l'envers*, or the other side, or the lining, of the discourse of the master. Lacan, J. (2007). *The Seminar of Jacques Lacan Book XVII: The Other Side of Psychoanalysis*. R. Grigg (Trans.). New York & London: W. W. Norton & Co.

across a church that has been recently destroyed—paradoxically, not by the choreography of renouncers and state but by a surplus, a bomb left over from another war in another time—and a cat's head amongst the rubble, its body dispersed by the explosion. She is moved by a poignant and urgent intensity of feeling. She takes up the head and wraps it in her handkerchief, compelled to find a place of green to lay it in. And suddenly, in his predatory way, the milkman is beside her, pointed like an arrow, like a gun—*Where are you going? What are you doing? What is the point? You must have a point. Jump in and I will appoint you*—pressing her, making her see her act diminished as a silly, girlish fancy. She can't escape, but she resists—embarrassed, girly, guilty as he makes her—until he leaves her alone in the night, no longer reading-while-walking but scared, vigilant, agitated. Then suddenly, real milkman is there, also with a van but a real milk van, and she gets in and speaks to him in her agitation, not of the milkman, whom throughout the book she speaks of only once and then mistakenly, but about the cat's head and the necessity of finding it a place. He says, "Will I take it off you?" and does, and places it in a velvet bag until it can be buried in a patch of green, as they agree.[39] He takes it not as an act of possession but in the spirit of completing her act: In this moment, they are one in transference, in trans. He has a " 'How can we get this done?' manner", she says, "not the prevalent 'What's the point, [. . .] it's not gonna make any difference [. . .]?'" manner. Real milkman, driving-while-listening, in continual movement, open to all voices, is able to be with her otherness.

It is a moment synonymous with the one in which an analysis begins or ends—an event; the emergence of an excess or of an order word, to use a term of Deleuze and Guattari.[40] A certain truth—perhaps it's been repressed, but does that matter?—stops not being written: not in that it's spoken, but in that it affects her, and then in that they are commanded to make an act together, in trans-ference. Real milkman *could* endow her act with meaning—he *could* interpret that she is mourning that aspect of her femininity which is rejected beyond the pale, called "cat" and defamed. He *could* translate the instant in which she is gripped and commanded by what she sees, into the Freudian instant of a girl's seeing and knowing what she is without. Such interpretations would be attempts to organ-ise her jouissance, to re-orient her sexuality to the phallus, to restore identity to her becoming. It would be to do what the milkman does to her. Real milkman doesn't do any of those things.

If psychoanalytic discourse brings the unknown knowledge of the unconscious to the status of truth, that truth is not a correspondence of one thing with another thing. It might rather be the singularity of a true act—the finding of a place of green to bury a cat's head—which is true only in one particular instant. Christian Fierens,

39 Burns, A. (2018). *Milkman*, p. 143.

40 For Deleuze and Guattari, an order word affects and commands; it brings about a change of state. There is a sense of immediacy, an instantaneous apprehension, not one which is built up by a series of propositions or representations. Deleuze, G. and Guattari, F. (2013). *A Thousand Plateaus*, pp. 118–128.

in his seminars given at the Freudian School of Melbourne, spoke of truth as a movement, an errancy rather than a fixity, a wandering-while-saying. If the truth that emerges in an instant from her perambulation can "fall onto the real", according to Lacan, it is only insofar as it *remains* impossible to represent, and real milkman can witness it only insofar as he doesn't translate it. He lets her love be what it is without making it the making-one of Eros. He takes her speech not as meaning but as *command*, and thus allows a knowledge which neither of them knows to be apprehended truthfully.

The therapist in me asks *And so? What then? What good does it do to merely receive or witness? How does it help?* Can you hear the echo of *What's the point? There's no point*—the sound of the pale closing? Being in discourse, I know, as each of us knows, how to be or play the man, to find the use value of speech, to reorgan-ise another's speech, to hunt down meanings and herd those wanderers back inside the pale, to take the other as my soul, to shore up my narcissism by knowing. That's the discourse one *is* in, the discourse of the master with its signification of the phallus.

That discourse is possible because it is preceded by a necessary point of *fixion*—or the fixing by language of a point in the real from which fiction can arise as truth. This first fixity is that of a name, what Saul Kripke called a rigid designator, what for Lacan was the Name of the Father, and whom Freud imagined as the Father of the primal horde, he who had the right to enjoy all the women.[41,42] In this novel composed of a plurality of voices and of ways of jouissance, the only rigid designator is *Milkman*—for, surprise! although he has been referred to all along as "the milkman", no-one knew why, it emerges after he is shot, to everyone's confusion, that "milkman" is not a descriptor but his proper name—*MILKMAN REALLY MILKMAN!* screams the newspaper headline after his death.[43] Milkman *is* the rigidity, the same-to-same, the identical-to-self which fixes a point in the real from which the phallic fiction can unfold; he is the dream or nightmare of the Father who knew all jouissance—which necessarily makes him, as Lacan points out, the dead father, a myth, the place of jouissance as lost or prohibited.[44]

Freud's myth tells us that the Father's death binds All the sons in a pact of incestuous prohibition by which the object they can have is a substitute for the one and only object which is prohibited, ceded, sacrificed. Desire follows loss and returns in its circuit not to the object but to the narcissism of possession. The discourse of the master, of the unconscious structured by this circuit, inherits the rigidity that designates the Father's name. It makes the Pale. For Freud, as for the town depicted in the novel, the problem is how to fit women into this circuit—or rather,

41 For Saul Kripke, a name is a rigid designator in that, in every possible world, it designates the same object. Kripke, S. (1972). *Naming and Necessity*. MA: Harvard University Press, p. 48.

42 Freud, S. (1913 [1912–1913]). Totem and taboo: Some points of agreement between the mental lives of savages and neurotics. SE XIII: 162.

43 Burns, A. (2018). *Milkman*, p. 323.

44 Lacan, J. (2007). *The Seminar of Jacques Lacan Book XVII*.

how to account for them accepting as subjects the position of object that the circuit assigns them. It is Lacan who observes that a woman is not-all, that her jouissance is not-all tied to the objectal circuit of desire but can also wander, solitary, un-fixed, non-designated—not a dark continent but a becoming-open to all the colours of the sunset.

If analysing is to maybe-open to the real beyond the pale of the master discourse, then, it could only be by *not* knowing, *not* grasping the point, *not* wielding the power of trans-lation, by receiving a truth that will not *be* identical to one's knowledge or even to itself, but will *be-coming*, an infinite and varied becoming which may occur in an instant or in a meandering that, in Irigaray's words, "upsets the linearity of a project, undermines the goal-object of a desire, diffuses the polarization towards a single pleasure, disconcerts fidelity to a single discourse".[45] If this is so, then there is no being-analyst but only becoming-analyst, in a shared instant of transference.

45 Irigaray, L. (1985). *This Sex Which Is Not One*. C. Porter and C. Burke (Trans.). Ithaca & New York: Cornell University Press, p. 30.

Chapter 16

The Winds

Fragment of a possible novel[1]

Sabina Spielrein

Translation and Introduction
Michael Gerard Plastow

Forty years have now transpired since the first publication of this curious text from the hand of Sabina Spielrein, written in French. It is an unusual piece, as it is the only indication that we have of Spielrein writing what is explicitly framed as a fragment of a novel, that is, an extended piece of prose fiction. It is unfortunately the only fragment that was found and known to exist of this "possible novel". In its content, it is explicitly framed as a division, or *Spaltung* to use Freud's term, in the experience of a protagonist who remains unnamed. There is a further division that Cifali comments upon in what follows, that of a division of languages in Spielrein's experience, since this is the third language in which she writes, after Russian and German. It is striking that Spielrein chooses this language to express herself in this creative form, even if, of course, this is the language of the place in which she was living at that time: Lausanne in Switzerland. We might say that Spielrein lives and writes her division.

This fragment was found by Mireille Cifali, who published it along with her Presentation of the text. It was located amongst the cache of papers left by Spielrein in Geneva in the hands of Edouard Claparède when she departed Geneva for her native Russia in 1923 and which were refound in 1975 by the Italian scholar Carlo Trombetta. Spielrein's German biographer Sabine Richebächer describes the format of the piece in the following manner: "The hand in which the characters of the diary are written now resembles scribbles: lines, words and phrases fly apart in all directions".[2] It is not clear exactly when Spielrein's piece was written, but it would seem to be between the years of 1915 and 1920.

"The Winds" was published in a French psychoanalytic journal in the early 1980s and followed soon after the publication in English in 1982 of the book *A Secret Symmetry: Sabina Spielrein between Jung and Freud* by Jungian analytical

1 First published as "Les Vents", by Sabina Spielrein, with a Presentation by Mireille Cifali. In: (1983). *Patio*, no. 1, 84–87.

2 Richebächer, S. (2005). *Sabina Spielrein: Eine fast grausame Liebe zur Wissenschaft*. Munich: btb Verlag, p. 208.

DOI: 10.4324/9781003712480-20

psychologist Aldo Carotenuto.[3] The latter's work contained excerpts of diaries and letters that were part of the same cache of documents discovered in Geneva in 1975, as well as Carotenuto's own sensationalised account of Spielrein's history, which included his claim that Spielrein had had a sexual relationship with Carl Jung, her analyst. In addition, in this book Carotenuto asserted that Spielrein was not just psychotic but schizophrenic to boot. His claim was no doubt in part designed to discredit Spielrein's stature as a theoretician of some notable significance, to Jung's benefit, endeavouring thus to salvage Carl Jung's reputation. Carotenuto's claim that Spielrein suffered from schizophrenia was echoed by Bruno Bettelheim in his Commentary in the 1983 edition of the same book, nominally giving it a broader credence.[4]

Despite the salacious bent to Carotenuto's claims being quite clear in retrospect, his story of Sabina Spielrein became something of an overnight hit. This would give rise to much wider echoes, fuelled as it was by derivative works such as John Kerr's *A Most Dangerous Method* and the play by the English playwright Christopher Hampton *The Talking Cure*, partly based upon Kerr's work.[5,6] Following on from these came the sexualised David Cronenberg film that was partly based on both of these, titled *A Dangerous Method.*[7] Less known perhaps to an English-speaking audience was the Italian film of a similar predilection titled *The Soul-Keeper*, which had the advantage, however, that it had a broader and more accurate historical sweep.[8] Carotenuto's book and his account of Sabina Spielrein's story and the works that followed this—rather than Spielrein's theoretical opus, which has remained relatively unknown—had a profound influence upon how her work would be received both within and without psychoanalytic circles. It remains the case that often, including among many analysts, the only thing known about Spielrein is what is portrayed through the prurient film *A Dangerous Method.*

Whilst most scholars today doubt the veracity of Carotenuto's claims, the story that has emerged from his misrepresentation of her history has nonetheless shaped the way that Spielrein's work is read and understood . . . or rather, mostly unread and misunderstood. In fact, the interest in her story has only increased, with the consequence that the attention to her theoretical work continues to be limited. Not all of her theoretical papers have been translated, and what translations exist are rather patchy, and many contain very significant errors, even concerning what papers have been attributed to her.

3 Carotenuto, A. (Ed.). (1982). *A Secret Symmetry. Sabina Spielrein between Jung and Freud*. New York: Pantheon.
4 Carotenuto, A. (Ed.). (1984). *A Secret Symmetry*. (Commentary by Bruno Bettelheim).
5 Kerr, J. (1993). *A Most Dangerous Method: The Story of Jung, Freud & Sabina Spielrein*. New York: Vintage.
6 Hampton, C. (2002). *The Talking Cure*. London: Faber & Faber.
7 Cronenberg, D. (Dir.). (2011). *A Dangerous Method*. Sony Pictures Classics.
8 Faenza, R. (Dir.). (2002). *Prendimi l'Anima* [The Soul Keeper]. Medusa Film.

How can we now read "The Winds" from Sabina Spielrein? We might also ask how we might read a dream or the play of a child in a session. No doubt the modality of our reading will determine what we might extract from it. Sabine Richebächer reads it as "the chronicle of a depression", in other words, something that invites her to give the author of the piece another diagnosis, even if it is not schizophrenia on this occasion.[9] She goes on to ask, "Is the author, with the 'landscapes devastated by the north-east wind', describing her own internal state, or is she speaking of her Russian homeland that is situated in the north-east and is being afflicted by a terrible war?" Richebächer seems to lean towards the latter hypothesis, as she goes on to write of the Great War, and in particular how four million Russian soldiers fell: dead, injured, imprisoned or lost.

Thus Richebächer emphasises a reference point outside Spielrein's text, specifically the external reality of the outside world. From psychoanalysis, however, in order to grasp the logic of a text, we do not require an a priori reference point outside it, whether it is the text of the speech of the analysand or, in this case, the letter of the text that is written here. This text has its own texture; indeed, it is a textile with its own warp and weft, elements that maintain a constant relation to each other. It is this very structure that we must endeavour to grasp.

In relation to this period in Lausanne, Renata Udler Cromberg—in the recently published second volume of her complete works of Sabina Spielrein in her native Portuguese—emphasises Spielrein's correspondence with Jung over this period. She cites Spielrein's response to Jung sending her his latest work, "The Psychology of the Unconscious Processes".[10,11] Thus, in her first letter of this period, Spielrein replies, "I read your book some time ago now and I would like to discuss many different things with you. This must be divided into a series of letters".[12] Here, Spielrein already begins through a necessary division. Udler Cromberg rightly stresses here the modality of Spielrein's transference to Jung. And indeed, in this correspondence, as I have commented elsewhere, there is effectively a failure of correspondence.[13] Spielrein certainly writes in transference, but I would propose that now she writes to her ex-analyst in a transference to work. As she foreshadows in the "many different things", Spielrein does not content herself to agree with the word of her former analyst and supervisor. On the contrary, she writes at length and utilises these letters in the production of the most explicit elaboration of her own theoretical apparatus in response to Jung's writings of that time. On the other hand,

9 Richebächer, S. (2005). *Sabina Spielrein*, p. 208.

10 Udler Cromberg, R. (Ed.). (2021). *Sabina Spielrein: Uma pioneira da psicanálise. Obras Completas*, vol. 2, R. Dias Mundt (Trans). São Paulo: Blucher.

11 Jung, C. G. (1917). *Psychologie der unbewussten Prozesse. Ein Überblick über die moderne Theorie und Methode der analytischen Psychologie*. Zürich: Verlag von Rascher & Cie.

12 Carotenuto, A. (Ed.). (1986). *Tagebuch einer heimlichen Symmetrie; Sabina Spielrein zwischen Jung und Freud*. Kore: Freiburg i. Br., p. 141.

13 Plastow, M. G. (2019). *Sabina Spielrein and the Poetry of Psychoanalysis*. Abingdon, Oxon: Routledge, p. 130.

Jung's letters tend to be quite brief and are often dismissive with a critical tone. His letters were not included in the English version of Carotenuto's book but were in the German. Jung does not in any way take up what we might consider to be the position of analyst but rather that of the one who knows. He writes, for instance, in returning a letter: "I have underlined in your letter all the places in which you think concretely, and typically misunderstand the symbol".[14]

Jung, in this correspondence, also underlines another division, that of the Christian and the Jew, here using this division to criticise Jewish people, Spielrein as well as Freud: "Do not forget that the Jew also had prophets . . . That is—'unfortunately'—the curse of the Jew: he calls the deepest and most private aspect of his soul 'infantile wish-fulfilment,' he is the murderer of his own prophets, even of his Messiah."[15] In this correspondence Spielrein also reminds Jung of her own long-standing division between psychoanalysis and music, a dichotomy that continues to divide her in Lausanne. She reminds Jung that he had told her that she would lose her mind if she allowed herself to make music.[16] For Spielrein, however, one side of this divide does not exclude the other: Again, she lives her division.

As we see in what follows, Mireille Cifali also comments upon Spielrein's own division in "The Winds". In reference to part of a journal published as "Unedited extracts from a diary" from 1906 or 1907, she reads the division in Spielrein's paper between the two winds as a division that is exemplified by a duality of two men: Carl Gustav Jung and Sigmund Freud.[17] She cites Jung's division of two psychological types, the introvert and the extrovert, as a division between Jung and Freud, a division between two positions that Jung endeavours to differentiate, but to also reconcile so that they do not mutually exclude each other.[18] Cifali, in introducing this, notes however that Spielrein,

> continues to be haunted by a duality: two winds, the one from the north-east and the other from the south. Her text, through its structure, strangely echoes that written by Jung in 1913, at the moment of his rupture with Freud.

We can also hear that even though this division is exemplified by Jung and Freud, it is nonetheless a division that presents itself in Spielrein and is articulated through her writing.

My reading of the split articulated in this diary extract referred to by Cifali is, effectively, the very same division that Spielrein experiences here in these

14 Carotenuto, A. (1986). *Tagebuch einer heimlichen Symmetrie*, p. 218.
15 Carotenuto, A. (1986). *Tagebuch einer heimlichen Symmetrie*, pp. 219–220.
16 Carotenuto, A. (1982). *A Secret Symmetry*, p. 72.
17 Spielrein, S. (1983). Unedited extracts from a diary (1906/1907?). P. Bennett and B. Wharton (Trans). In: *Journal of Analytical Psychology*, 2001, p. 46.
18 Jung, C. G. (1913). Contribution à l'étude des types psychologiques. Communication présentée au Congrès Psychanalytique de Munich, 1913. *Archives de Psychologie*, T. XIII, Nr. 53. Déc. 1913.

subsequent writings. In "The Winds", both positions are articulated in a masculine voice—or rather, we can say, a neutral voice—the voice of the non-sexed subject of psychoanalysis. In the diary extract the division is articulated as a discourse between two "speakers", of whom the first, who "reaches the summit of his art only when he gives himself up to passion", is herself as the south wind. The other speaker who possesses "a logical spirit, derisive, playful but nonetheless terrible",[19] is easily identified as Jung and the north-east wind. These two voices are, nonetheless, but two aspects of a single discourse, we might even say two deities—Dionysus and Apollo—in one godhead. In other words, there are two "speakers", but there is only one speech that Spielrein articulates in this diary. There are two voices or two winds, two breaths. And one's wind—for instance, in the expression "long-winded"—is indeed defined as breath, the breath that is utilised in speaking. Wind or breath is also *psyche* in ancient Greek, the breath being inextricable from life and the soul, in other words from the life of the subject itself. We should note that Spielrein, like Freud, uses the German word for soul, *Seele*, when she refers to the subject.

The division into two winds also takes us back to Spielrein's 1913 paper, "Destruction As Cause Of Becoming", in which she states, "I had to reach the insight that the principal characteristic of the individual consists in the fact that it is a dividual".[20] Spielrein indeed grasps that she as subject is divided, and the division is experienced in this short text here in the form of these two winds. And Spielrein has the knack of being able to theorise this division not as an ego—it is not hers personally—but rather that of the subject of psychoanalysis. This division of the subject elaborated here by Spielrein also anticipates Lacan's later formulation that the subject is divided by language. The subject—which only exists within language and through language—is divided by language in the same manner as these "winds".

Here, it is only possible to sketch out an overview of a reading of the text. A reading to the letter might also demonstrate, at least in the French, that the title "Les Vents", is a quasi-homophone for the Levant, the east, which might give rise to yet another wind. And the word for the north-east wind that blows across Lake Geneva used here by Spielrein is *la bise*, also a homophone for "kiss" in French. In the concluding paragraph of this short text, Spielrein refers to *la bise*, and in the very next line, this resonates with the word "brisent", or "break". Hence, through the use of rhyme, Spielrein counterposes the unity of the north-east wind with the division enacted by the commotion of the South Wind. Such further readings to the letter of the translation of the text, from this point onwards, must be left to the reader.

19 Jung, C. G. (1913). Contribution à l'étude des types psychologiques, p. 156.

20 Spielrein, S. (1912). Die Destruktion als Ursache des Werdens. In: *Jahrbuch für psychoanalytische und psychopathologische Forschung*, vol. 4, no. 1, pp. 465–503, 471.

Spielrein, Sabina. "Les Vents". Patio, No. 1, 1983

Presentation by Mireille Cifali

Sabina Spielrein wrote this sketch of a future novel in French in one of her black notebooks in which she was accustomed to inscribe the fragments of her thought. In this notebook, there are other fragments of a diary, composed in German, and whose dates are those of 1916 and 1919.

Sabina Spielrein must have put this Chapter X down on paper while she was living in Lausanne, or even later in Geneva, where she became the registrar [*assistant*] of Edouard Claparède at the Jean-Jacques Rousseau Institute and a psychoanalyst responsible for analysing the people of Geneva, who were considered dilettantes by Freud.

In 1923, returning to Russia quite certainly due to financial reasons, Sabina consigned all her precious documents to Edouard Claparède: personal diaries of her adolescence, love letters, correspondence with her family. This legacy remains enigmatic to this day. Why did she not take these testimonies of her existence with her, she for whom this was no longer a first migration? Why did he not have the opportunity to return them to her? This fragment of a future novel was part of this legacy in abeyance [*en souffrance*] in the city of Calvin. It is currently in possession of Edouard Claparède's descendants.

"The Winds" was thus written in a hesitant French. We have retained the significant errors, such as the one that made Spielrein put an "s" in without passions. It is necessary to emphasise that as far as we know, French is the third language spoken by this young woman after Russian, her mother tongue, and German, the language of her psychoanalysis.

Whether this chapter was composed in 1916 or 1919 matters little to us. It comes after an upheaval, but as Spielrein indicates to us, as a woman, she continues to be haunted by a duality: two winds, one from the north-east and the other from the south. Through its structure, her text provides an echo to that written by Jung in 1913, at the moment of his rupture from Freud. Carl Gustav Jung had read "Contribution to the Question of Psychological Types" at the Munich Congress, but he very quickly published it, in French, in the Genevan *Archives de Psychologie*.[21] There are, according to Jung, two types: the introvert and the extrovert, which he desperately endeavours to differentiate, but also to reconcile so that they do not mutually exclude each other. Thus there would be two, represented in an exemplary manner by himself and Freud.

Sabina Spielrein chooses the Southern Wind, the breath of the depths, against logic, intelligence and desiccation. She seems to continue to be inhabited by passion and death, creation and the dread of a mystery that has vanished. Her novel is nonetheless written in the masculine. I [*Je*] is masculine. Is there a fault in the agreement of gender in her French, or can we hear in this another signification?

21 *Archives de Psychologie*, Volume XIII, 1913.

In any case, she does not cease from being between-two [*entre-deux*], she who fertilised the thought of two men, that of Jung and that of Freud.[22]

Fragment of a possible novel

Chapter X "The Winds"

For five days the north-east wind [*la bise*] had raged, cantankerous and impetuous. The sky was an implacable shade of grey. In truth more grey than blue, although not a single cloud put in an appearance. A grey with no beauty, an indefinable and oppressive grey. The north-east wind had raged, cantankerous and impetuous, sweeping away all the poetry that this late autumn of setting suns had left behind. Like the clear intelligence of a man born for action, or of a rigorous logician, the north-east wind systematically set aside the sentimental naïveté of mists and the painful beauty of the last purple leaves.

But to us, life seemed morose and cold, without passion[s], organised and clear. But now, during the night the north-east wind suddenly dropped, like a haughty knight who falls from his mount at the edge of a forest, unhurt but struck down by some violent and furtive harm to the bewildered eyes of his companions.

And this morning, upon waking, we had the impression of being plunged into a warm and perfumed bath. We felt released from an invisible vice around our heads. The air was suddenly pleasant to breathe. It was a halt following a strenuous march. The sweetness of clear water at our tired feet.

The north-east wind suddenly dropped like a fallen warrior, and it was then that we perceived that this warrior was a tyrant and that his death gave us back our freedom. We felt free and released from all servitude. Free like the young man who has just broken up with his mistress, free like the artist who confronts life . . .

Then, everything changed.

The lake took on a dark tinge and began to stir. The sky filled with marvellous clouds. Red appeared once again in the countryside, nature began to dream once more. One could see that autumn was not yet dead, and its attractive and profound charm is that of a young consumptive woman who distances herself from the very illness that gives her such a soft hue, and her noble languidness that deliciously sharpens her most voluptuous desires.

The south wind is a colossal Shakespeare that one thought one had seen, judged and filed away. One believed that one had experienced it all, and suddenly one is alarmed to see that everything can be different.

Passion, or greatness of character, transforms the most common things into ardent novelties.

The south wind carries passion and a whole world of fecund dreams.

22 Spielrein, S. (1983). Unedited extracts from a diary (1906/1907?), p. 156. First published in French in *Bloc-Notes de la psychanalyse*, no. 3, 1983.

The north-east wind had said to us: 'I am the truth, I clear the mists from the summits, I clarify, I organise'.

The south wind tells us: 'I am the most profound truth, my heavy clouds are our lively passions, the air that I make you breathe is filled with marvellous possibilities, with fiery dreams. I am life. The north-east wind is nothing but a critic and I am a great artist. I make the landscape in my image, tormented and grandiose. The north-east wind only dissects things, it creates nothing'.

"Oh South wind, you are the image of my passionate heart".

Now, I was sad from too much thinking. I had felt the futility of all effort, and I was weary. Action seemed ridiculous to me, and dreams useless. I was sad and discouraged. The perfidious north-east wind had strangely desiccated my spirit. The sky of my thought was a bleak grey. My despair held no beauty, since beauty is made of mystery. Mystery was dead.

You come, oh South Wind, and I see that you alone are true, that you alone create and incite creation. The chimaera of your heavy clouds is a hundred times more true than the impoverished clarity of landscapes devastated by the north-east wind. The commotion of the waters that you drive out and that break in their tragic effort is that of my bruised heart. You carry dreams, illusions, and mystery along with you and it is for that reason that you alone are true, since you create, oh South Wind, and you incite creation. And yet to live is to create. And whoever no longer creates is already dead.

Part V

Translation of *Ou il y a symptôme et sinthome* by Jean Allouch

Chapter 17

Introduction to the translation of *Où il y a symptôme et sinthome* by Jean Allouch

Tine Nørregaard

This paper was presented at the conference A Tribute to the Work of Cormac Gallagher in Dublin from November 30 to December 1, 2018. Peter Gunn brought the paper back from the conference with a suggestion to translate it into English and to invite a discussion of the paper in the work of the Freudian School of Melbourne. We then contacted Jean Allouch, who generously gave permission to translate the paper. It appears here both in the original French version and in the English translation. Sadly, Jean Allouch passed away in September 2023, and the appearance here of this paper both in French and in English is also a way for the School to pay homage to him, by continuing to produce a work from each of our transferences to his writings.

The work of translation of the paper evolved as the work of a Cartel, which produced in itself a separate discourse evoking questions about the work of translation in a school of psychoanalysis and questions opened by the reading of Jean Allouch's paper. The work of the Cartel produced the writing of three separate papers, which also appear here.

DOI: 10.4324/9781003712480-22

Chapter 18

Où il y a symptôme et sinthome

Jean Allouch

Ce titre est d'abord un constat: les deux termes se trouvent chez Jacques Lacan, le second lui étant, pourrait-on dire, comme apporté par James Joyce le Dublinois. De ce constat résulte un problème élémentaire que signalent trois questions convergentes. S'agirait-il d'une substitution telle que « sinthome » aurait mis fin à « symptôme » ? Ou bien d'une seule et même essence qui se laisserait approcher de deux différentes façons ? Ou, plutôt, y aurait-il là deux différents concepts qui devraient être soigneusement distingués ? Auquel cas un des problèmes soulevés pourrait être celui de leur cohabitation, voire de leur articulation.

Cette troisième option me paraît devoir être retenue, et je me propose donc de vous soumettre les raisons de ce choix. M'y a conduit ce qu'il m'est arrivé récemment d'isoler chez Lacan, à savoir la discrète présence de deux différentes « analytiques du sexe », la première focalisée sur l'objet *a*, la seconde sur l'inexistence du rapport sexuel. Et ce sont donc ces deux différentes analytiques du sexe que je me dois de vous présenter tout d'abord, afin de jeter, de là, quelque lumière sur la distinction du symptôme et du sinthome. Cela me semble convenir au regard de ces deux journées en hommage à Cornac Gallager où l'on s'interroge sur deux différents symptômes, l'un dit « de groupe », l'autre singulier. Est-ce envisageable que ce dernier puisse s'appeler « symptôme » tandis que le premier relèverait du « sinthome » ?

Répondre ne sera possible qu'en présentant trois points:

1) les deux analytiques du sexe;
2) la sexuation de l'Autre;
3) la raison qui contraint à différencier symptôme et sinthome.

On les abordera selon une méthodologie commune, car ce à quoi renvoie le nom de Jacques Lacan, ce ne sont pas des « cours » (Jacques-Alain Miller), pas tant non plus des énoncés, ni des mathèmes, mais des *parcours*; ils sont composés d'énoncés et de mathèmes, mais qui varient et qui ne peuvent donc être lus qu'en envisageant leurs cheminements, leurs variations, leurs transformations. Varité, mieux que vérité.

DOI: 10.4324/9781003712480-23

Deux differentes analytiques du sexe

Cette différenciation m'est apparue nécessaire tout d'abord du fait d'un énoncé qui m'a troublé, heurté, choqué et ainsi mis au travail. Il se laisse ranger dans la liste des propos tenus par Lacan qui se démarquent de la suite que l'on attendait. On conjecturait une explicitation, un développement, une prolongation, et l'on se trouvait confronté à un pas de côté qui, souvent, portait silencieusement atteinte au savoir prétendument acquis. Ce qui eut lieu des milliers de fois. Voici donc une de ces déclarations *déplacées* (au sens où un propos est « déplacé », malvenu) dite le 26 janvier 1975 en réponse à une question de Marcel Ritter: « Il y a un rapport avec le sexe en ceci que le sexe est partout là où il ne devrait pas être; il n'y a pas, nulle part, de possibilité d'établissement en quelque sorte formulable du rapport entre sexes. »

Qu'entendre par « le sexe est partout où il ne devrait pas être » ? Que, là où il est, croit-on, il n'est pas à sa place, pas en place, ou encore qu'il *ne tient pas en place*—un peu comme on le dit d'un enfant agité. Le sexe est *dévoyé*, déporté hors de son chemin. Or, en n'étant pas en son lieu, qui plus est en étant logé là « où il *ne devrait pas* être », le sexe n'est plus lui-même, cela au point que Lacan pourra un beau jour déclarer, sans plus aucun souci de Freud, que la sexualité est une « défense » (25 janvier 1967). Le sexe ne serait lui-même qu'en se tenant à sa place. Déplacez le premier violon loin de sa place à la gauche du chef d'orchestre, mettez-le « là où il ne devrait pas être », par exemple au beau milieu des cors, il s'ensuit une cacophonie: la musique ne se joue ni ne s'entend plus.

L'énoncé de 1975 « le sexe est partout où il ne devrait pas être » n'aurait pas été concevable si Lacan n'avait antérieurement déclaré (4 juin 1969): « Il n'y a pas de rapport sexuel. » En envisageant le sexe en tant que rapport, il fit *ipso facto* valoir un inédit registre du sexuel, tout à la fois différent et voisin de celui qu'à la suite de Freud il avait jusque-là étudié et reconfiguré. Depuis cette déclaration du 4 juin 1969 une version *unitaire* de l'érotique analytique n'était plus tenable. Jacques Lacan était loin d'être le seul à avoir ainsi *distribué* l'érotique, quoiqu'il l'ait fait d'une façon à nulle autre pareille. Je m'en tiendrai à vous présenter en un tableau quelques-uns de ces auteurs, et non des moindres, qui, eux aussi, ont scindé l'érotique selon deux registres[1]:

	Registre 1	*Registre 2*
Platon	Désir sexuel	Érotique métaphysique
Lacan	Analytique de l'objet *a*	Analytique du rapport sexuel
Foucault	Dispositif de sexualité	Dispositif d'alliance
Rubin	Sexe	Genre

1 Dans *Pourquoi y a-t-il de l'excitation sexuelle plutôt que rien ?* (Paris, Epel, 2017) j'ai présenté l'ensemble des données qui ont rendu possible leur formalisation dans ce tableau.

Le « domaine spécifique » que constitue la seconde analytique du sexe n'est pas signalé par le seul énoncé « il n'y a pas de rapport sexuel ». Deux autres « il n'y a pas » convergent avec celui qui porte sur le rapport sexuel: « Il n'y a pas d'Autre de l'Autre » et « Il n'y a pas de jouissance de l'Autre ». Ces trois énoncés sont liés, car s'il y avait un Autre de l'Autre, on pourrait toujours se demander, ayant admis que l'Autre ne jouit pas, si l'Autre de l'Autre ne serait pas, lui, susceptible de jouir. Et nul ne doute que l'absence de cette jouissance de l'Autre concerne au plus près le rapport sexuel qui, quoique inexistant, ne cesse de solliciter cette jouissance qui s'avère absente à chaque rendez-vous que l'on croyait lui avoir fixé. Ainsi ces trois inexistences sont-elles assignables à une seconde analytique du sexe, celle du traumatisant parce que inexistant rapport sexuel. Qui plus est, Lacan les a logées sur une même plage d'un nœud borroméen mis à plat, une plage qu'il affirme être celle du « vrai trou », qui n'est donc pas celle où il inscrivait petit *a* (la distinction des deux analytiques est ici *écrite*):

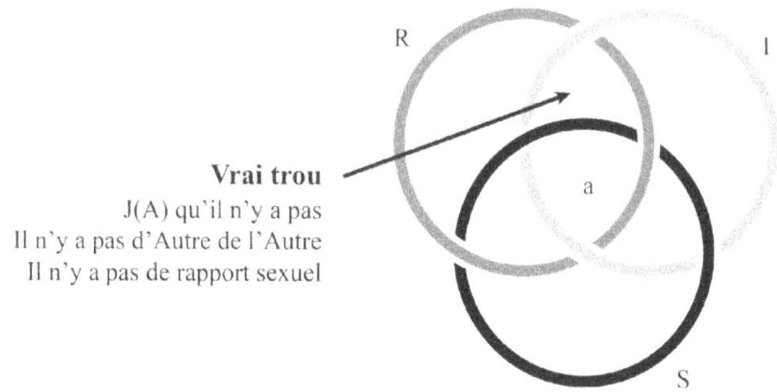

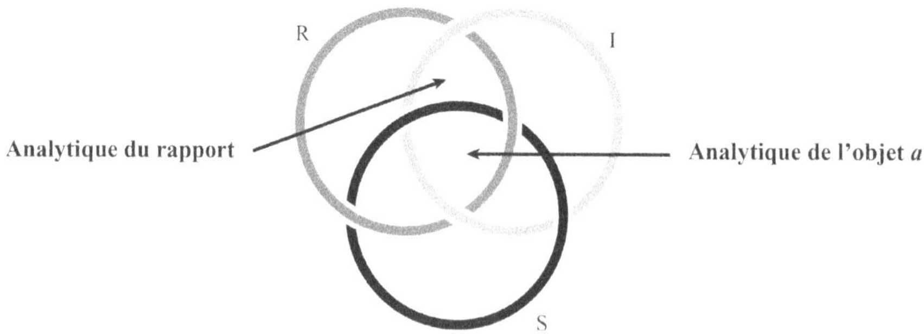

Sexuation de l'Autre

La conception selon laquelle l'Autre pourrait sexuellement jouir n'apparaît guère convenir si on l'entend depuis la première définition de l'Autre comme « trésor des signifiants ». Elle devient moins étrange si l'on note la transformation que Lacan fit subir à son concept de grand Autre—avec, toutefois, une constante: cet Autre fut d'emblée pensé comme l'*Autre que soi*, non pas l'*Autre de soi*, ce dernier ouvrant largement les bras à la psychologie tandis que le premier, conforme en cela au Dieu des chrétiens, s'en dispense.

Rappel: cet Autre fut, un temps, conçu comme un Autre sujet. Selon cette perspective reconnue comme « intersubjective », le sujet ne peut advenir qu'au lieu de cet Autre sujet. Ainsi l'inconscient a-t-il été défini comme « discours de l'Autre », le désir vu comme « désir de l'Autre », le fantasme écrit avec l'objet petit *a* logé au lieu de l'Autre, l'auto-érotisme a été porté au compte, non d'un soi-même, mais d'un manque de soi.

Avoir d'abord voulu son Autre « trésor des signifiants » posait un problème: où donc se trouvait ce trésor ? Son lieu ne saurait simplement être un pur réceptacle sans aucune incidence sur ce qu'il contient. Cela tient au fait que *la place* assignée au signifiant intervient dans la détermination de la signification. Tel est le cas, par exemple, de notre numérotation de position, où 1 suivi de 2 a une autre valeur que 2 suivi de 1. Ou encore: un blanc-bec n'est pas un bec blanc. Ainsi l'Autre fut-il toujours plus pensé comme lieu—ledit « lieu de l'Autre ». Première étape qui, déjà, mettait à mal l'intersubjectivité.

Nouveau pas de cette métamorphose de l'Autre: ce lieu, qu'une topologie fit valoir en tant que surface, cette surface, donc, est corporéisée. Le lieu de l'Autre, est-il dit en 1967 (*La Logique du fantasme*), n'est « pas à prendre ailleurs que dans le corps ». S'ensuivit, six ans plus tard, un nouveau et ultime pas où ce corps est reconnu sexué:

> « L'Autre dans mon langage, ce ne peut être que l'Autre sexe » (1973, Encore). J'ai cru pouvoir écrire en un seul mot: « Autresexe » et explorer la portée de ce terme tout au long d'un récent ouvrage.[2]

Cet Autre d'abord fait trésor, puis lieu, puis corps, puis sexe[3] n'était-il pas spécialement bien fait pour être pris comme partenaire d'un rapport sexuel ? Corps sexué, il pourrait jouir. Autresexe, sa place paraît toute trouvée dans un rapport sexuel vu comme « une relation définissable comme telle entre le signe du mâle et celui de la femelle » (4 juin 1969)—cela d'autant plus aisément que, en français classique tout au moins, l'expression « autre sexe » équivalait à « féminin ».[4]

2 *L'Autresexe*, Paris, Epel, 2015.

3 Autant de qualifications qui ne s'excluent pas l'une l'autre, tandis que les faire simplement cohabiter pose problème.

4 *Le Trésor de la langue française* cite Renan: « Pour la fille, il [le vicaire] avait ces manières réservées qu'ont nos ecclésiastiques bretons avec les "personnes du sexe", comme ils disent » (*Souvenirs d'enfance et de jeunesse*, 1883, p. 32). On disait de Molière qu'il avait « un penchant pour le sexe », ce que tout un chacun comprenait aisément, ce que l'espagnol désigne d'un terme qui n'a aucun équivalent en français: « *mujeriego* ». Dans ses *Caractères* (1880), La Bruyère écrit: « L'honnêteté,

Or, *voilà exactement le pas à ne pas franchir*. La jouissance de l'Autre « reste en suspens », ou encore « à la dérive » (14 juin 1967). Et, surtout, *voilà le point clé, la pierre d'angle qui rend nécessaire que l'érotique soit distribuée en deux différentes analytiques*. Une seule aurait « suffi » si l'Autre jouissait. Lacan ferme cette porte maintenue grande ouverte par le catholicisme avec son « *fruitio Dei* » (jouissance de Dieu).

Par touches successives et discrètes, Lacan va étayer la distinction de ces deux analytiques. Ainsi, le 4 février 1973, déclarait-il: « Cet objet petit *a*, [. . .] ce n'est pas l'Autre, ce n'est pas l'Autre sexe, c'est l'Autre du désir. » L'Autresexe est ici distingué d'un Autre du désir. Une analytique de petit *a* (de la pulsion, du fantasme, de l'angoisse, du désir) est à différencier de celle de l'inexistant rapport sexuel. Le désir causé par *a* tient à un Autre de désir maintenant différencié de l'Autresexe (ainsi est-il mis fin à ce que j'appellerai « l'impérialisme du désir de l'Autre »); il relève de la loi sexuelle, désormais, reconnue anormale, alors même qu'elle concerne tout un chacun.

La mise en question du désir vu, avec Hegel, comme « désir de l'Autre » apparaît on ne peut plus claire dans une déclaration de 1967, postérieure, donc, à la trouvaille de petit *a*: « Si "le désir de l'homme c'est le désir de l'Autre", il arrive qu'il faille bien que son désir à l'homme soit le sien propre.[5]»

La même année, ce n'est rien de moins que la conception freudienne de la libido qui se trouve piquée au vif: « [. . .] ce qui s'articule dans la théorie psychanalytique moderne en long et en large, la confusion de cet Autre nourricier avec cet Autre sexuel » (18 janvier 1967). La formidable trouvaille freudienne de la *libido*, concept apparu chez Augustin[6] et regroupant toutes les excitations de quelque ordre pulsionnel qu'elles soient, est ici mise à mal.

Symptome et sinthome

Tel un papillon émergeant de sa chrysalide, comment le sinthome a-t-il pu naître et s'émanciper du symptôme ? Voici, dessiné à grands traits, quel fut ce parcours où une continuité débouche sur une séparation.

Avec Sigmund Freud, l'analyse a conçu le symptôme autrement que ne le faisait la psychiatrie de son temps. Freud découvrait que la contracture hystérique renvoyait à un souvenir traumatique,[7] et Lacan que la folie de Marguerite Anzieu

les égards et la politesse des personnes avancées en âge de l'un et l'autre sexe me donnent bonne opinion de ce qu'on appelle le vieux temps. » Il n'y a nulle ambiguïté non plus dans ce titre d'un ouvrage de Margaret Mead: *L'un et l'autre sexe*.

5 Dans « Place et origine de mon enseignement ».

6 « *Excepterum me consolationes lactis humani* [. . .] post et ridere coepi. » avait écrit Augustin, *Confessions*, I, 6 (7–8): « Et m'ont recueilli les consolations du lait humain [. . .] Plus tard, j'ai commencé à rire. »

7 Un traumatisme conçu fort différemment que chez Charcot, dissocié des zones innervées du corps et lié à ce que le langage opère de découpage des corps.

témoignait d'une problématique qui lui venait bel et bien de son histoire (qu'il ne s'agissait donc pas d'un

« processus psychique[8] »). Chez l'un et l'autre, l'historisation du symptôme prend le dessus sur sa localisation médicale au sein d'une entité clinique qu'il serait censé composer avec d'autres, ses semblables.[9] Il a fallu du temps, toutefois, pour que certains analystes, dont je suis, délaissent la psychopathologie.

Ainsi historiquement situé, le symptôme pouvait être traité (*Durcharbeitung*) et, pour finir, céder. Il devient sans objet lorsque, en parlant à quelqu'un, sont mises au jour, perdant ainsi de leur virulence, les tensions érotiques propres à une histoire qui n'en finissait pas de ne pas finir. Ce schéma était séduisant, il a séduit: la disparition du symptôme prouvait sa validité.[10]

Toutefois, c'était ne pas compter avec ce que l'on allait bientôt découvrir et dénommer « transfert ». Entreprendre une analyse modifie d'emblée la situation où l'on se trouve et que l'on souhaite changer. Un personnage nouveau (« la personne du médecin », selon cette expression freudienne récurrente sur laquelle Guy Le Gaufey a attiré l'attention) est introduit dans l'intimité du sujet et au sein de son réseau relationnel. Cela a lieu au présent, en présence, et a fini par apparaître plus décisif que l'histoire. On découvrait, surpris, que certains patients pouvaient fournir au médecin tel ou tel symptôme, simplement parce qu'il était su que ce médecin s'y intéressait. Et aussi qu'à elle seule la « mise en acte de l'inconscient », autrement dit le transfert (Lacan), pouvait mettre fin au symptôme,[11] ce que l'inverse, d'ailleurs, vérifiait: une interruption brusque du transfert pouvait donner lieu à une recrudescence du (ou des) symptôme(s). À cet égard, un des cas les plus exemplaires, quoique hors exercice analytique, fut publié par Pierre Janet. Pauline Lair Lamotte devient délirante *le jour même* où meurt ce Père Conrad[12] qui supportait son transfert en validant son engagement extrême, elle, une riche bourgeoise, dans la charité évangélique auprès des plus pauvres parmi les pauvres.

8 Un des combats livrés par Lacan dans sa thèse de 1932 a consisté à écarter la conception de la psychose comme processus pour faire place à la réaction. Je discute ce point dans *Marguerite, ou l'Aimée de Lacan*, Postface de Didier Anzieu [1990], 2e éd. revue et augmentée, Paris, Epel, 1994.

9 L'architecture alors à l'œuvre était la suivante: symptôme, syndrome, entité clinique, maladie.

10 Il fut pris au sérieux et vivement contesté par Adolf Grünbaum (*La Psychanalyse à l'épreuve*, trad. de l'angl. (USA) par Joëlle Proust, Paris, Éd. de l'éclat, 1993; *Les Fondements de la psychanalyse, une critique philosophique*, trad. de l'angl. par Jean-Claude Dumoncel et révisé par Élisabeth Pacherie, Paris, PUF, 1996). J'ai proposé une lecture critique de cet ouvrage dans « Adolf Grünbaum lecteur de Freud: d'une juste critique en porte à faux » (*L'Unebévue*, n° 10, automne/hiver 1997, pp. 73–100).

11 Certains parmi les premiers psychanalystes étaient au désespoir d'avoir affaire à une disparition à leurs yeux trop précoce des symptômes car, disaient-ils, elle permettait au patient d'éviter l'analyse.

12 Cf. Jacques Maître, *Une inconnue célèbre. La Madeleine Lebouc de Janet*, Paris, Anthropos, 1993. Mon commentaire dans « Du symptôme comme tenant hypothétiquement lieu de sainteté », *Littoral*, n° 41, novembre 1994, pp. 53–64.

Et voici qu'il est arrivé quelque chose à cette personne du médecin support du transfert et partie prenante de sa résolution. Lacan, en 1973, ne prétend à rien de moins que de la « situer objectivement ». Il est, déclare-t-il, « ce qui dans le passé s'est appelé: être un saint[13] ». Qu'est-ce à dire ? Le texte le précise: il fait le déchet, il« décharite »; ne jouissant pas, il est le rebut de la jouissance, ouvrant ainsi au sujet la possibilité de le prendre pour la cause abjecte de son désir.
Conclura-t-on de tels propos relèvent de l'analytique de l'objet *a* ? Luther vient à l'esprit: « Nous sommes les étrons tombés de l'anus de Dieu.[14]» Cependant, cette plongée lacanienne dans la sainteté est porteuse d'autre chose que de la seule opération séparant l'objet *a* et grand A—il s'agit de « charité » chez Luther, de « décharitér » (un verbe, un acte) chez Lacan. Ainsi soupçonne-t-on déjà que le symptôme pourrait relever de la première analytique et le sinthome de la seconde.

Ce qui se confirmera bientôt. Moins de deux ans après avoir fait de l'analyste un saint, la sainteté viendra frapper de son sceau le symptôme, avec l'exhumation de la première orthographe de ce mot: *sinthome*. De l'un à l'autre, du *saintanalyste* au sinthome, Joyce aura été un joint, peut-être même décisif.[15] La conférence « Joyce le symptôme » est du 16 juin 1975[16]; sa transcription comporte six occurrences du terme« sinthome », deux d'entre elles étant « Joyce le sinthome », cela en dépit du titre qui a élu « symptôme » et non pas « sinthome ».[17] Notamment celle-ci: « Joyce le sinthome fait homophonie avec la sainteté, dont quelques personnes ici peut-être se souviennent que je l'ai télévisionnée. »
L'homophonie alors constatée ne renvoie à aucune identité. Joyce le sinthome n'est pas déclaré être un saint, notamment pas un saintanalyste. Et pas non plus un symptôme car, que l'on sache, un symptôme n'a pas de nom propre, or c'est ainsi que Lacan procédait: offrir son nom propre de « Joyce le sinthome » à un James Joyce qui n'en aurait sans doute pas voulu.

« Joyce le sinthome » est quelqu'un. Il en ira de même lorsque Lacan donne corps à deux figures respectivement dénommées « sinthome-il » et « sinthome-elle » afin de recueillir « tout ce qui reste de ce qu'on appelle le rapport sexuel », un rapport dès lors reconnu « intersinthomatique ».[18] Tout au long du séminaire Le

13 Jacques Lacan, *Télévision*, Paris, Éd. du Seuil, 1973, p. 28.

14 Dans d'autres occurrences, il s'agit non pas de Dieu mais d'une de ses créatures: le diable. On peut voir sur Internet une gravure de Cranach l'Ancien représentant la situation presque inverse: Luther déféquant dans la tiare du pape: http://jackaimejacknaimepas.blogspot.com/2017/05/la-defecation-de-luther.html

15 On pourra se reporter aux pages que je consacre à ce problème dans *La Scène lacanienne et son cercle magique. Des fous se soulèvent*, Paris, Epel, 2017, p. 164 sq.

16 Six mois plus tard vient la première séance du prochain séminaire préalablement annoncé avec pour titre *Le Sinthome*.

17 On verra dans ce flottement terminologique l'indice d'un problème non résolu. « Sinthome » disparaît dans la version écrite de la conférence, parue en 1979.

18 Fait rarissime, la chose est dite par deux fois à l'identique, tout d'abord le 9 juillet 1978 en conclusion d'un congrès de l'École freudienne, puis le 22 octobre de la même année, dans une intervention intitulée « Pour Vincennes ».

Sinthome, plusieurs personnages d'un théâtre d'ombres vont venir occuper cette même place où se joue l'inexistence du rapport sexuel: saint Thomas d'Aquin, tout d'abord,[19] ainsi que la figure du père (18 novembre 1975); l'autre sexe, ensuite, ici défini comme « celui auquel je n'appartiens pas » (17 février 1976) et, pour finir, le psychanalyste (13 avril 1976).

Il ne reste, me semble-t-il, plus aucun doute: le sinthome est à inscrire dans l'analytique du rapport sexuel. Tous deux reconnus comme sinthomes, Joyce et l'analyste jouent différemment leur partie. Tel que le décrit Lacan, Joyce est un maître, pas un saint. Son œuvre, faite d'un langage sphérique, autrement dit non troué, promeut son nom propre.[20] Il en va différemment avec l'analyste qui, parce que lui aussi est un personnage incarnant le sinthome et parce que son exercice n'est pas fait pour promouvoir son nom, peut, de là, permettre que son rapport intersinthomatique avec l'analysant (ce qui fut appelé « transfert ») se boucle sur l'inexistence de cet Autresexe et celle du rapport sexuel, autrement dit sur le caractère troué du langage, troué par cette inexistence même (l'impossibilité d'écrire le rapport sexuel).

Du groupe psychanalytique

Ne serait-ce pas dans le jeu de cette intersinthomatique que devrait être situé ledit symptôme de groupe ? Sans en avoir épuisé les ressorts, je crois avoir fait plus d'un pas dans le sens d'une réponse affirmative à cette question. Il s'ensuit que l'on devrait plutôt écrire « sinthome de groupe ». Toutefois, les problèmes rencontrés par les groupes psychanalytiques relèvent-ils du seul sinthome ? Il ne semble pas possible d'écarter que des transferts non bouclés trouvent à se prolonger dans la vie des groupes. Le registre de tels transferts est, lui aussi, d'ordre intersinthomatique et le groupe peut jouer comme un point d'appel pour ces transferts « suspendus » (d'autant que des psychanalystes ne reculent pas user de cette corde en assignant un rôle dans leur groupe à des analysants par eux élus—Lacan, lui aussi, l'avait cru possible et pratiqué[21]).

Envisager certains des problèmes rencontrés dans les regroupements analytiques à partir de l'analytique du rapport pourrait permettre d'orienter les inévitables décisions que tout groupe doit prendre concernant aussi bien sa composition que son fonctionnement. On se demandera alors: comment configurer ce fonctionnement de façon qu'il ne fasse pas obstacle à l'accès de chacun à l'inexistence du rapport sexuel ? Une telle question n'a rien d'abstrait, elle concerne aussi bien 1) le statut lui-même du groupe (association, cercle, école, etc.); 2) le mode selon lequel s'y

19 Une homophonie, là encore: sinthom . . . adaquin.

20 Je déplore le caractère lapidaire de ces derniers propos et ne peux, ici, que renvoyer à *La Scène lacanienne et son cercle magique, Des fous se soulèvent*, Paris, Epel, pp. 163–179, où la position de Joyce le sinthome est présentée et discutée.

21 Analysant, je ne lui ai laissé aucune possibilité d'agir de même avec moi.

prennent les décisions; 3) l'admission dans le groupe; 4) le dispositif de la passe; 4) les cartels.

Lacan jugeait décisive cette dernière question, celle des cartels. En avril 1975, lors d'une « Journée des cartels[22] », fut largement discuté ce qui avait été posé comme« plus un », ou encore « plus une personne », différente en cela des trois autres membres du cartel (chiffre minimum pour que soit composé un cartel, le maximum étant six). Certains tenaient à ce que cette « plus une personne » soit quelqu'un; d'autres le voulaient aussi, mais faisaient de ce « plus une » une fonction tournante parmi les membres du cartel. Ce choix signalait une crainte, à savoir que cette « plus une personne » exerce une chefferie, cela au nom d'une prétendue expérience plus assurée et d'un savoir plus certain, ces deux traits étant admis par les membres du cartel.

En 1975, prenant exemple sur les mathématiciens chez lesquels, affirmait-il, la mathématique elle-même est une personne, Lacan écartait toute chefferie en proposant que la psychanalyse soit cette « plus une personne ». En ouvrant largement la porte à ce qui s'est appelé un « transfert latéral », le choix de la chefferie tient à bonne distance les membres du cartel de l'inexistence du rapport sexuel; celui du plus une personne incarnée par l'analyse n'y fait pas obstacle. L'analyse, elle seule, peut trancher si un énoncé est recevable ou s'il doit être écarté.

22 *Lettres de l'École freudienne*, n° 18, avril 1976.

Chapter 19

Where there is symptom and sinthome

Jean Allouch

This title is first of all an observation: The two terms are to be found in Lacan, the second as if it were brought to him by James Joyce the Dubliner. From this observation comes an elementary problem that indicates three convergent questions. Is it a question of a substitution in which "sinthome" had done away with "symptom"? Or is it a question, rather, of one and the same essence that could be approached in two different ways? Or might there be two different concepts that should be carefully distinguished? In which case one of the problems raised could be that of their cohabitation, even their articulation.

It seems to me that this third option must be retained, so I propose to submit to you the reasons for this choice. What led me to this is what I have recently been able to isolate in Lacan, that is, the subtle presence of two different "analytics of sex," the first focused on the object *a*, the second on the inexistence of the sexual relation. So it is these two different analytics of sex which I must present to you in order to throw some light from this onto the distinction of the symptom and the sinthome. This seems to me to be suited to these two days of homage to Cormac Gallagher, where we are examining the two different symptoms, one said to be of the "group," the other singular. Could we envisage that the latter might be called "symptom" while the first would pertain to the "sinthome"?

It will only be possible to answer by presenting three points:

1 The two analytics of sex
2 The sexuation of the Other
3 The reason that constrains us to differentiate symptom and sinthome

We will approach these according to a common methodology, because what we are referred to by the name of Jacques Lacan are not "courses" [*cours*] (Jacques-Alain Miller), nor are they statements, nor mathemes, but *trajectories* [*parcours*]; they are composed of statements and mathemes but which vary and which can therefore only be read by considering their progressions, their variations, and their transformations. Varity [*varité*], better than truth [*vérité*].

DOI: 10.4324/9781003712480-24

Two different analytics of sex

This differentiation seemed necessary to me first of all because of a statement that troubled, jolted, and shocked me, thus putting me to work. It can be placed in the list of remarks, made by Lacan, that stood out from the sequel that was expected of them. We speculated about an explanation, a development, an extension, and found ourselves confronted by a side step that, often, infringed silently upon the knowledge that had supposedly been acquired. This happened thousands of times. Here is one of these *misplaced* [*déplacé*] declarations (in the sense that a remark is "misplaced," unwelcome) articulated 26 January 1975 in reply to a question from Marcel Ritter:

> There is a relation with sex in so far as sex is everywhere it should not be; there is not, anywhere, the possibility of establishing, in any manner that can be formulated, the relation between sexes.[1]

What is to be understood by "sex is everywhere it should not be"? To believe that, wherever it is, it is not in its place, not in position, or even that it *does not stay in place*—a little like one might say of a restless child. Sex is led astray, *delinquent*, borne off its course. And yet by not being in its place, being lodged moreover "where it *should not be*," sex is no longer itself, to the point that Lacan is able to declare one fine day, with no longer the slightest concern for Freud, that sexuality is a "defence" (25 January 1967).[2] Sex would only be itself by remaining in place. Move the first violin far from its place on the left of the orchestra conductor and place it "where it should not be," for example right in the middle of the horns, and there follows a cacophony: the music is no longer played nor heard.

The statement of 1975, "sex is everywhere it should not be," would have been inconceivable if Lacan had not previously declared (4 June 1969): "There is no sexual relation."[3] By considering sex as a *relation*, he highlighted, *ipso facto*, a completely new register of the sexual, at the same time both different and akin to

1 There may be an error here in the French of Allouch's paper, given that there does not seem to have been a session of January 26, 1975, in Lacan's seminar of 1975–1976. There is a session of January 21, 1975, in which Lacan discusses the symptom at length. Unfortunately, questions from the audience and Lacan's answers are not recorded in the two English-language versions consulted. See Lacan, J. (1982). *The Seminar of Jacques Lacan Book XXII R.S.I. 1975–1976*. C. Gallagher (Trans.). Non-commercial edition; and Mitchell, J. and Rose, J. (Eds.). (1982). Seminar of 21 January 1975. In *Feminine Sexuality. Jacques Lacan and the école freudienne*. New York & London: W. W. Norton & Co., 162–171. [Ed.].

2 Lacan, J. (1966–1967). *The Seminar of Jacques Lacan Book XIV The Logic of Phantasy 1966–1967*. Unpublished manuscript. [This reference and subsequent references to English language editions of the *Seminars*, are to give a reference for Anglophones. Allouch, of course, was quoting from a French manuscript. We have given a translation of his words. (Ed.).].

3 Lacan, J. (1968–1969). *The Seminar of Jacques Lacan Book XVI From an Other to the Other*. C. Gallagher (Trans.). Non-commercial edition.

the one that, following Freud, he had studied and reconfigured up to that point. Following this declaration of 4 June 1969, a *unitary* version of the erotic analytic was no longer tenable. Jacques Lacan was far from being the only one who had *distributed* the erotic in this way, although he did it in a manner without equal. I would like to present to you, in a table, some of these authors, and not the least of them who have also divided the erotic between two registers:[4]

	Register 1	*Register 2*
Plato	Sexual desire	Metaphysical erotics
Lacan	Analytic of the object *a*	Analytic of the sexual relation
Foucault	Device [*dispositif*] of sexuality	Device of alliance
Rubin	Sex	Gender

The "specific domain" that constitutes the second analytic of sex is not indicated just by the statement "there is no sexual relation." Two other "there is no" converge with the one that bears the sexual relation: "There is no Other of the Other" and "There is no jouissance of the Other." These three statements are tied, because if there were an Other of the Other, one could always wonder, having accepted that the Other does not enjoy [*ne jouit pas*], whether the Other of the Other is not prone to enjoying [*de jouir*]. And no one doubts that the absence of this jouissance of the Other very closely concerns the sexual relation, which, despite being inexistent, does not cease to solicit this jouissance which proves to be missing at every rendez-vous we thought we had made with it. Thus these three inexistences are assigned to a second analytic of sex, that of the traumatising-because-inexistent sexual relation. Lacan, moreover, lodged them on the same beach as a Borromean knot laid flat, a beach that he claims is that of the "true hole," which is thus not the one where he inscribed the little *a* (here the distinction between the two analytics is *written* [*écrite*]):

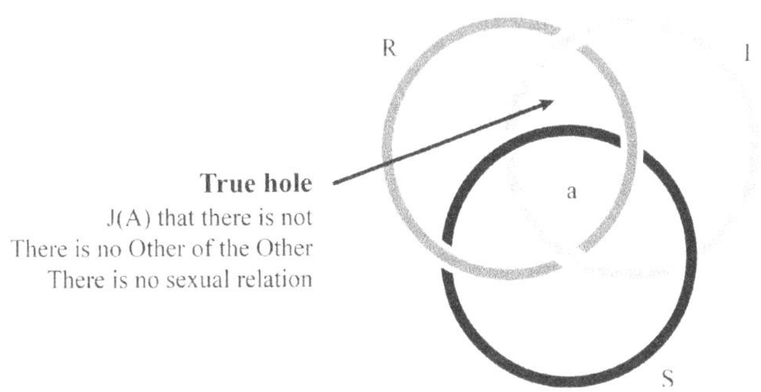

4 In Allouch, J. (2017a). *Pourquoi y a-t-il de l'excitation sexuelle plutôt que rien?* Paris: Epel. I have presented all the elements which made possible their formalisation in this table.

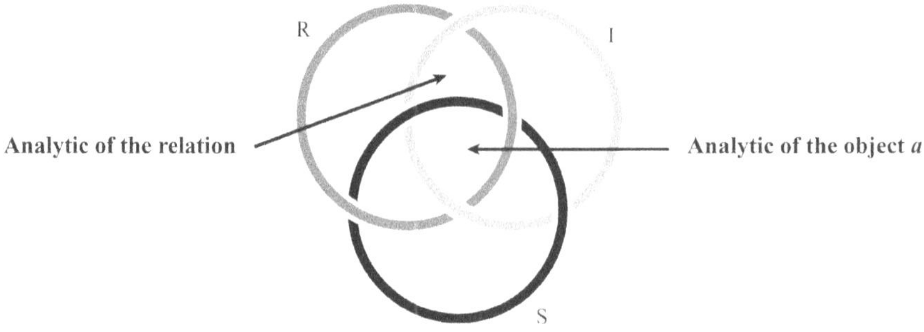

Sexuation of the Other

The conception according to which the Other might be able to sexually enjoy [*jouir*] hardly seems to be suitable if we understand it according to the first definition of the Other as "treasury of signifiers." It becomes less strange if we note the transformation to which Lacan subjected his concept of the big Other—with, however, one constant feature: This Other was, first of all, considered as *Other than oneself,* not *Other of oneself*, the latter opening its arms widely to psychology while the former, in the model of the God of the Christians, dispenses with it.

A reminder: This Other was, for some time, conceived of as an Other subject. According to this perspective, accepted as "intersubjective," the subject can only appear in place of this Other subject. Thus the unconscious was defined as "discourse of the Other," desire seen as "desire of the Other," the fantasm written with the object little *a* [*petit a*] lodged in the place of the Other, the auto-eroticism being brought to the account not of a self but of a lack of self.

Having from the start wanted his Other to be a "treasury of signifiers" posed a problem: Where, therefore, was this treasure to be located? Its place could not simply be a pure receptacle without any effect on what it contains. This is due to the fact that *the place* assigned to the signifier intervenes in the determination of the signification. Such is the case, for example, with our numbering of position, where 1 followed by 2 has a value other than 2 followed by 1. Or again: a greenhorn [*blanc-bec*] is not the same as a green horn [*bec blanc*]. Thus the Other was always thought of more as place—the so-called place of the Other. This is the first step that, already, puts intersubjectivity into trouble.

A new step is this metamorphosis of the Other, this place that a topology highlighted as surface, and this surface, thus, is made corporeal. The place of the Other, as was said in 1967 (*The Logic of the Fantasm*), is not "to be taken otherwise than in the body."[5] There followed, six years later, a new and final step in which this body is recognised as sexuated: "The Other, in my language, can only be the Other

5 Lacan, J. (1966–1967). *The Seminar of Jacques Lacan Book XIV*.

sex" (1973 *Encore*).[6] I believed I could write in a single word: "Othersex," and explore the scope of this term throughout a recent work.[7]

Was this Other, first made treasury, then place, then body, then sex, not especially well suited to be taken as partner of a sexual relation?[8] A sexuated body can enjoy. The place of the Othersex seems to be all located in a sexual relation, viewed as "a relation, definable as such, between the sign of the male and that of the female" (4 June 1969)—all the more easily since, in classical French, the expression "other sex" was more or less equivalent to "feminine."[9,10]

Now, this is exactly the step [*le pas*] that must not be taken. The jouissance of the Other "remains in suspense," or again, "adrift" (14 June 1967).[11] And above all, this is the key point, the cornerstone which makes it necessary that the erotic be distributed in two different analytics. One alone would have "sufficed" if the Other enjoyed. Lacan closes this door held wide open by Catholicism with its "fruitio Dei" (jouissance of God).

By successive and discrete touches, Lacan will shore up the distinction of these two analytics. Thus, on 4 February 1972, he declared: "This object little *a* . . . it is not the Other, it is not the Other sex, it is the Other of desire."[12] The Othersex is distinguished here from an Other of desire. An analytic of little *a* (of the drive, of the fantasm, of anguish, of desire) is to be differentiated from that of the inexistent sexual relation. The desire caused by *a* is attached to an Other of desire now differentiated from the Othersex (thus an end is put to what I would call "the imperialism

6 Lacan, J. (1998). *On Feminine Sexuality, the Limits of Love and Knowledge 1972–1973. Encore the Seminar of Jacques Lacan Book XX*. J.-A. Miller (Ed.), B. Fink (Trans.). New York & London: W. W. Norton & Co.

7 Allouch, J. (2015). *L'Autresex*. Paris: Epel.

8 These are so many qualifiers that are not mutually exclusive, whereas to simply make them coexist would be problematical.

9 Lacan, J. (1968–1969). *The Seminar of Jacques Lacan Book XVI*.

10 *Le Trésor de la Langue Francaise* cites Ronan: "For the girl, he [the vicar] had these reserved manners that our Breton ecclesiastics have with 'persons of the sex,' as they say." [Renan, E. (1883). *Souvenirs d'enfance et de jeunesse*. Paris: Nelson Éditeurs, p. 32. Allouch has made a slip of the pen in the name of this author. (Ed.).].

[The *Trésor de la langue française* is a 16-volume dictionary of 19th- and 20th-century French published by the Centre de Recherche pour un Trésor de la Langue Française from 1971 to 1994. (Ed.).].

It is said of Molière that he had "a penchant for the sex," which anyone and everyone easily understood; what is designated in Spanish by a term that has no equivalent in French: "*mujeriego*" [womaniser]. In his *Caractères*, La Bruyère writes: "The honesty, the consideration and the politeness of persons of advanced age of one and the other sex give me a good opinion of what is called the olden days." [De la Bruyère, J. (2018 [1688]). *Les Caractrères de la Bruyère*. Sydney: Wentworth Press.]

Neither is there any ambiguity in the title of a work of Margaret Mead: *L'un et l'autre sexe*. [This is the title given to the French translation of Mead's *Sex and Temperament*. Mead, M. (1977 [1935]). London: Routledge and Kegan Paul. (Ed.).].

11 Lacan, J. (1966–1967). *The Seminar of Jacques Lacan Book XIV*.

12 The relevant session of Lacan's seminar . . . *Ou Pire* seems, in fact, to have taken place on 9 February. Lacan, J. (1971–1972). *The Seminar of Jacques Lacan Book XIX . . . Ou Pire/. . . Or Worse 1971–1972*. C. Gallagher (Trans.). Non-commercial edition. (Ed.)].

of the desire of the Other"); it is a matter of the sexual law, henceforth recognised as abnormal, even when it concerns each and every one.

The putting into question of desire that is seen, with Hegel, as "desire of the Other" can be no more clearly perceived than in a declaration of 1967, posterior, therefore, to the discovery of little *a*: "If 'the desire of man is the desire of the Other,' it happens that it would indeed be necessary that the desire of man be his very own."[13]

The same year, it is nothing less than the Freudian conception of libido which is cut to the quick: "what is articulated at great length in modern psychoanalytic theory, the confusion of this nutritive [*nourricier*] Other with this sexual Other" (18 January 1967).[14] The formidable Freudian discovery of the *libido*, a concept which appeared in Augustine and gathered together all the excitations, of whatever order of the drive they may be, here comes to harm.[15]

Symptom and Sinthome

Like a butterfly emerging from a chrysalis, how has the sinthome been able to be born and become emancipated from the symptom? Here, roughly sketched, is what made this trajectory in which a continuity gives rise to a separation.

With Sigmund Freud, analysis conceived the symptom otherwise than was done by the psychiatry of his time. Freud discovered that hysterical spasm referred to a "traumatic memory," and Lacan that the madness of Marguerite Anzieu attested to a problematic that well and truly came to her from her history (that it was not, therefore, a matter of a "psychical process").[16,17] In the one and the other, the historicisation of the symptom gets the upper hand over its medical localisation within a clinical entity that it would be supposed to constitute with others, its fellows [*semblables*].[18] It has required some time, however, for certain analysts, myself among them, to abandon psychopathology.

13 In "Place et origine de mon enseignement." [The full title is "Place, origine et fin de non enseignement." https://ecole-lacanienne.net/wp-content/uploads/2016/04/1967-00-00.pdf. Publication in English: The Place, Origin and End of My Teaching. In Lacan, J. (2009). *My Teaching*. J.-A. Miller (Ed.), D. Macey (Trans.). Brooklyn, NY: Verso. (Ed.)].

14 Lacan, J. (1966–1967). *The Seminar of Jacques Lacan Book XIV*.

15 "*Excepterum me consolationes lactis humani [. . .] post et ridered coepi*" Augustine had written, *Confessions*, I, 6 (7–8): "And my having received the consolations of human milk [. . .] Later, I started to laugh."

16 A trauma conceived of very differently than by Charcot, dissociated from the innervated zones of the body and tied to what language operates in cutting up bodies.

17 One of the battles brought by Lacan in his thesis of 1932 consisted in separating the conception of psychosis as process in order to make place for reaction. I discuss this point in Allouch, J. (1994). *Marguerite, ou l'Aimée de Lacan*. Postface by Didier Anzieu (1990). Paris: Epel, 2nd ed. revised and augmented.

18 The architecture of the work at the time was the following: symptom, syndrome, clinical entity, illness.

Thus, historically situated, the symptom was able to be treated (*Durcharbeitung*) and, finally, to give way. It becomes devoid of object when, while speaking to someone, the erotic tensions belonging to a history that would not stop not finishing are brought to light, thus losing their virulence. This schema was seductive, it has seduced: The disappearance of the symptom proved its validity.[19]

This did not, however, take account of what we were soon going to discover and name "transference." To embark upon an analysis, from the very beginning, modifies the situation that one finds oneself in and that one wishes to change. A new character ("the person of the doctor," according to this recurring Freudian expression to which Guy Le Gaufey has drawn attention) is introduced into the intimacy of the subject and the heart of his relational network. This takes place in the present, in presence, and has ended up appearing more decisive than the history. It was discovered, surprisingly, that certain patients had been able to furnish the doctor with such-and-such a symptom simply because it was known that the doctor was interested in it. And also that only the "putting into play of the unconscious," in other words the transference (Lacan), could put an end to the symptom, which was, moreover, verified by the opposite: An abrupt interruption of the transference could give rise to a recrudescence of the symptom(s).[20] One of the most exemplary cases in this regard, although outside of analytic practice, was published by Pierre Janet. Pauline Lair Lamotte became delusional *the very day* of the death of this Father Conrad who supported her transference by validating her extreme engagement, rich bourgeoise that she was, in the evangelical charity among the poorest of the poor.[21]

And then something happened to this person of the doctor, support of the transference, and party to its resolution. Lacan, in 1973, aspired to nothing less than "objectively situating" him. He is, Lacan declared, "that which in the past was called: being a saint."[22] What is he saying by that? It is specified in the text: He becomes the refuse, he "de-charitises"; by not enjoying [*jouissant*]; he is the reject of jouissance, thus for the subject opening up the possibility of taking him as the abject cause of his desire.

19 It was taken seriously and keenly contested by Adolf Grünbaum ((1993). *La Psychanalyse à l'épreuve*. J. Proust (Trans. to Eng.). Paris: Ed. de l'éclat.; (1996). *Les Fondements de la psychanalyse, une critique philosophique*. J.-C. Dumoncel (Trans. to Eng.), E. Pacherie (revision). Paris: PUF, 1996). I proposed a critical reading of this work in Allouch, J. (1997). Adolf Grünbaum reader of Freud: A sound critique gone astray. In: *L'Unebévue*, no. 10, automne/hiver 1997, pp. 73–100.

20 Some of the first psychoanalysts were in despair at being faced with what they viewed as a too-precocious disappearance of symptoms because, they said, it allowed the patient to avoid the analysis.

21 *Cf* Maître, J. (1993). *Une inconnue célèbre. La Madeleine Lebouc de Janet*. Paris: Anthropos. My commentary is in Allouch, J. (November 1994). Du symptôme comme tenant hypothétiquement lieu de sainteté. In: *Littoral*, no. 14, pp. 53–64.

22 Lacan, J. (1973). *Télévision*. Paris: Seuil, p. 28.

Can we conclude that such remarks concern the analytics of the object *a*? Luther comes to mind: "We are the turds fallen from God's anus."[23] This Lacanian plunge into sainthood, nonetheless, is the bearer of something other than just the operation separating the object a and big A—with Luther, it is a question of "charity"; with Lacan, it is a question of "de-charitising" (a verb, an act). Thus we already suspect that the symptom might be a concern of the first analytics and the sinthome of the second.

This would soon be confirmed. Less than two years after having turned the analyst into a saint, sainthood would come to strike its seal upon the symptom, with the exhumation of the first spelling of this word: sinthome. From one to the other, from the saintanalyst to the sinthome, Joyce was to be a bridge, perhaps even a decisive one.[24] The lecture "Joyce the sinthome" is from 16 June 1975; its transcription carried six occurrences of the term "sinthome," two of them being "Joyce the sinthome" despite the title in which Lacan had chosen "symptom" and not "sinthome."[25,26] And notably the following: "Joyce the sinthome is homophonic with sainthood, regarding which some people here might recall that I televisioned it."

The homophony thus noted refers to no identity whatsoever. Joyce the sinthome is not declared to be a saint, in particular not a saintanalyst. And not a symptom either since, as far as we know, a symptom does not have a proper name, and yet it is in that way that Lacan proceeded: by offering his proper name of "Joyce the sinthome" to a James Joyce who certainly would not have wanted it.

"Joyce the sinthome" is someone. The same applies when Lacan gives body to two figures respectively named "sinthome-he" and "sinthome-she" in order to gather together "all that remains of what can be called the sexual relation," a relation henceforth recognised as "intersinthomatic."[27] All through the seminar The Sinthome, several figures from a shadow theatre would come to occupy this same place where the inexistence of the sexual relation is played out: Saint Thomas Aquinas first of all, as well as the figure of the father (18 November 1975); next the

23 On other occasions, it is no longer a question of God but of one of his creatures: the devil. One can see on the internet an engraving by Cranach the Elder illustrating the almost-opposite situation: Luther defaecating into the pope's tiara. At: http://jackaimejacknaimepas.blogspot.com/2017/05/la-defecation-de-luther.html.

24 The pages that I dedicated to this problem can be referred to in Allouch, J. (2017b). *La Scène lacanienne et son cercle magique. Des fous se soulèvent.* Paris: Epel, p. 164 ff.

25 Six months later, the first session of the following seminar took place, provisionally announced with the title The Sinthome.

26 In this terminological wavering, we can see the indication of an unresolved problem. "Sinthome" disappears in the written version of the lecture, which appeared in 1979.

27 An extremely rare occurrence, this thing was said twice, identically, firstly on 9 July 1978 in concluding a conference of the Freudian School, then on 22 October of the same year, in a paper entitled "For Vincennes."

other sex, here defined as "the one to whom I do not belong" (17 February 1976), ending up with the psychoanalyst (13 April 1976).[28,29]

There remains, it seems to me, no longer any doubt: the sinthome is to be inscribed in the analytics of the sexual relation. Both recognised as sinthomes, Joyce and the analyst play their parts differently. As Lacan describes it, Joyce is a master, not a saint. His work, made of a spherical language, in other words not holed [*non troué*], promotes its proper name.[30] It is a different question in regard to the analyst who—because he is also a character who incarnates the sinthome, and because his activity is not made to promote his name—can, from that, allow his intersinthomatic relation with the analysand (what was called "transference") to be looped upon the inexistence of this Othersex and that of the sexual relation, in other words upon the holed nature of language, holed by this very inexistence (the impossibility of writing the sexual relation).

Regarding the psychoanalytic group

Would it not be in the play of the intersinthomatics that the aforementioned symptom of the group should be situated? Without having exhausted its mainspring, I believe I have taken more than one step in the direction of an affirmative answer to this question. It follows that we should instead write "group sinthome." Nonetheless, could the problems encountered by psychoanalytic groups pertain to the sinthome alone? It does not seem possible to rule out the possibility that some unlooped transferences manage to be extended into the life of groups. The register of such transferences is also of an intersinthomatic order, and the group can play the role of a point of appeal for those "suspended" transferences (all the more so since psychoanalysts do not hesitate to use such means by assigning a role within their group to analysands chosen by them—Lacan also believed this to be possible and practised it).[31]

To envisage certain problems encountered in analytic groupings from the perspective of the analytics of the relation could permit the orientation of the inevitable decisions of any group, whether they concern its composition or its functioning. We will ask ourselves then: How can this functioning be configured in such a way that it does not become an obstacle to each one's access to the inexistence of the sexual relation? There is nothing abstract about such a question, it concerns just as much: (1) the very status of the group (association, circle, school, etc.); (2) the

28 Here once again, is a homophony: sinthom . . . adaquin [Saint Thomas d'Aquin].

29 Lacan, J. (1975–1976). *The Seminar of Jacques Lacan Book XXIII Joyce and the Sinthome*. C. Gallagher (Trans.). Non-commercial edition.

30 I lament the terse character of these last remarks, and here, I can only refer the reader to Allouch, J. (2017b). *La Scène lacanienne et son cercle magique*, pp. 163–179, in which the position of Joyce the sinthome is presented and discussed.

31 As an analysand, I did not leave him any possibility of acting with me in this manner.

modality according to which decisions are made within it; (3) the admission into the group; (4) the device [*dispositif*] of the passe; (5) cartels.

Lacan considered the latter question, that of cartels, to be the decisive one. In April 1975, on the occasion of a "Colloquium of cartels," there was a lengthy discussion of what had previously been proposed as "plus one," or even "plus one person," different in this to the three other members of the cartel (the minimum number for a cartel to be formed, the maximum being six).[32] Some held this "plus one person" to be someone; others also wanted this but made the "plus one" a rotating function among the members of the cartel. This choice indicated a fear, that is, that this "plus one person" would exercise a leadership in the name of a supposed greater experience and a more certain knowledge, these two traits being accepted by the members of the cartel.

In 1975, taking the example of mathematicians among whom, he asserted, mathematics itself is a person, Lacan ruled out all leadership by proposing that psychoanalysis be this "plus one person." By leaving the door wide open to what was called a "lateral transference," the choice of leadership holds the members of the cartel at a good distance from the inexistence of the sexual relation; that of the plus one person incarnated by analysis does not constitute an obstacle to this. Only analysis itself can decide if a statement is admissible or if it must be ruled out.

32 Lettres de l'École Freudienne, No. 18, April 1976.

Part VI

Cartel on the translation of *Où in y a symptôme et sinthome*

Chapter 20

Introducing the cartel on the work of translation of *Où il y a symptôme et sinthome* by Jean Allouch

Tine Nørregaard, Michael Gerard Plastow, and Megan Williams

The work of translation of Allouch's paper put us to work from transference: a transference to the working of Lacan's concepts, a transference to Allouch's writing, a transference beyond each of our own analyses and the theorising that has come from this, a theorising that also forms different transferences of work in the School. The work of translation in psychoanalysis is a work of suffering, a jouissance that is worked in writing, and is an effect of this writing, in the way that Lacan spoke about the subject coming into being *en souffrance*, through a suffering, a suspense, a gap that is opened by the weight of the letter.[1] In considering our work of translation from the function of a cartel, each of us made a commitment to speak about how the weight of this work affected us; that is, to speak about the particular impact of the transference of work for each of us.

In our work, we each took charge of an initial translation of one part of the text, then each of us did a cross-over reading of one of the other translated parts. This was followed by a discussion between all of us that provided various suggestions for the translation of certain concepts and passages which we found difficult. During this working and reworking of the translation, we attempted to open these difficult concepts and passages by coming at them from different angles and thereby enabling new suggestions for the translation. This is a work which makes of a translation something that is evolving, not final. The rhythm of working and reworking formed our discourse of the translation of the paper and committed each of us to a project of writing. The three separate papers produced in this way were presented by each of us at the Seminar of the Freudian School of Melbourne on May 4, 2019. It is curious how these papers crisscross each other, maybe in the way that the wake of one boat intersects with the wake of another or the ripples of various stones thrown in a pond at the same time cross each other.

1 Lacan, J. (1966 [1956]). Le Séminaire sur "La Lettre Volée". In: *Écrits. Le champ freudien collection dirigée par Jacques Lacan*. Paris: Éditions du Seuil, p. 29.

DOI: 10.4324/9781003712480-26

Chapter 21

The plus one and the intersinthomatic of transference

Tine Nørregaard

For me, this work of translation has raised a central question: How can this be a work of a psychoanalytic school, that is, in conjunction with how the discourse produced in the school acts as a plus one for the cartel? This question concerns the transference as it continues from the analysis and charges the work in the psychoanalytic school and the group.

My early readings of Lacan's seminars in the psychoanalytic group in Denmark of which I was a member at the time often also involved the translation of the seminar as part of the work. Translation from one language to another has continued as the presence of an otherness in my transference of work in the Freudian School of Melbourne, an otherness that addresses an elsewhere beyond the School. I consider such a foreignness in the transference for each one as an important opening to an otherness in the discourse of psychoanalysis that is produced in the Freudian School of Melbourne. Lacan designated the plus one as the element that charges the transference and the work of the cartel.[1] Allouch notes in his paper that Lacan in 1975 ruled out any question of the plus one element being a leadership by asserting that the plus one is psychoanalysis.[2] This in effect means that it is from the transference in relation to the particular discourse of psychoanalysis that is written in each school that the work is produced. The plus one for our cartel puts us to work from each of our particular transferences to psychoanalysis and to Allouch's paper in the discussions of how to translate a particular concept, and this opened the possibility of it being a proper psychoanalytic translation that partakes in the work of the School.

The loopings of the transference and the sinthome

I will now consider a point in the translation that brought me to work. It concerns the discussions we had around the translation of the term "*se boucle*," which we

1 Lacan, J. (1990 [1964]). *Television: A Challenge to the Psychoanalytic Society*. J Copjec (Ed.), J. Mehlman (Trans.). New York & London: W. W. Norton & Company, p. 97.

2 Allouch, J. (2026 [2024]). *Where There Is Symptom and Sinthome*. In: *The Papers of the Freudian School of Melbourne. Lacanian Psychoanalytic Writings: The Littoral Word*. T. Nørregaard, M. G. Plastow and M. Williams (Trans.), M. Williams (Ed.). London: Routledge, vol. 27.

DOI: 10.4324/9781003712480-27

have translated as "being looped."[3] Allouch uses this term in relation to the transference that continues from the end of an analysis as the sinthome. He considers his transference which he names as intersinthomatic as being looped on the inexistence of the sexual relation. As he states, the analyst, like Joyce, is "a character who incarnates the sinthome," however, not in order to promote his name but to

> allow his intersinthomatic relation with the analysand (what was called "transference" to be looped upon the inexistence of this Othersex and that of the sexual relation, in other words upon the holed nature of language, holed by this very inexistence (the impossibility of writing the sexual relation).[4]

During our discussion, I considered whether we might translate "*se boucle*" with "to be knotted," and Michael made a reference to Lacan's use of the term *boucle* in the introduction to the French version of *Écrits*.[5] Here, the French term is translated from the English poem by Pope, *The Rape of the Lock*, as the lock or loop of hair that is secretly taken.[6] According to Lacan, this charming loop refers us to the topological sense of the word: a knot [*noeud*] whose trajectory is closed through its inverse redoubling, which is also what supports the structure of the subject as a divided subject.[7] So, in fact, there is a reference to a form of knot where the loop is a folding that falls back onto itself. This is a loop like the one of the Möbius strip where the subject and the object *a*, even if they are on the same plane, are found to be on opposite sides of the strip.

In the French edition of the seminar Sinthome, Lacan also uses the term *boucle* to designate the particular loopings in the Borromean knot of the real, the symbolic and the imaginary.[8] Here, this term refers to the manner in which the three registers are in fact completely separate and only form a knot through the looping of each one around the two others.[9] Lacan describes this by referring to cords that are infinite, where each one only finds itself looped with respect to the two other cords. I understand that this is an important point Lacan makes about the three registers which only form a knot through the loopings that sustain them as separate, in the sense that if one is cut, then all of them are freed. It is also through the particular Borromean looping of the rings that he asserts that there is no initiation of the subject. The three registers are not tied to a given reality which the subject can be

3 Allouch, J. (2026 [2024]). *Where There Is Symptom and Sinthome*.
4 Allouch, J. (2026 [2024]). *Where There Is Symptom and Sinthome*.
5 Lacan, J. (1966). *Écrits. Le Champ Freudien collection dirigée par Jacques Lacan*. Paris: Éditions du Seuil, p. 10.
6 Lacan, J. (1966). *Écrits. Le Champ Freudien collection dirigée par Jacques Lacan*.
7 Lacan, J. (1966). *Écrits. Le Champ Freudien collection dirigée par Jacques Lacan*.
8 Lacan, J. (1975–1976). *Le Sinthome. Séminaire 1975–1976*. Éditions de l'Association Freudienne Internationale, 2001. Publication hors commerce [non-commercial edition], session of 09.12.75.
9 Lacan, J. (1975–1976). *Le Sinthome*.

brought back to in analysis; the subject is always only supposed.[10] The division of the subject is an effect of language, and it is this division that constitutes the real, which means that this supposition is always open to an ambiguity. The Oedipus complex refers us to the function of the symptom as a knot that is particular to each one in accordance with how the three registers are looped. Lacan considers the sinthome as a different way of writing the symptom that, for Joyce, functioned as an artifice through his writing.[11] The sinthome is similar to the fourth term of the Borromean knot which is the additional loop that is woven around each of the three rings and hereby provides consistence to each of the rings. According to Lacan, it is this additional loop which enables the knot to continue as a chain, that is, to continue as a writing.[12] I am reminded that in his seminar *RSI*, Lacan also considers one more such element, written here as "+1," about which he asserts that if you subtract this, then there is no longer any chain.[13] According to Lacan, the sinthome functioned for Joyce as a subjective support through his art of writing, which, as he states, "replaced his phallic armour."[14] The sinthome sufficed for Joyce as something in the Other that was for him, as Lacan states, "charged from the father" (*chargé du père)*, so that a symptom was not required.[15]

I understand that Allouch's point of the intersinthomatic that is looped on the inexistence of the sexual relation also poses a question about how the Other is situated in the fantasm and the transference at the end of an analysis. We can say that this question addresses the way in which the transference that continues from the analysis is looped around the "traumatising-because-inexistent" sexual relation.[16] This looping does not prevent one from being affected by the anxiety of the jouissance of the Other that had underwritten the particular fantasm, but it is an anxiety which nevertheless comes from realising that there is no Other of the Other. As Allouch stresses, we are not without being confronted with a jouissance each time we cross paths with this impossible sexual relation, but it is an encounter that is always missed. This encounter with the traumatising-because-inexistent sexual relation which doesn't stop not being written nevertheless necessitates a writing, as the sinthome, as a new way of writing the symptom in the transference that continues from the end of an analysis. This additional loop of the transference evokes a writing from the lack in the Other, from having found a way to do with the lack imposed by the hole in the real where there is no order of existence.

10 Lacan, J. (1975–1976). *Le Sinthome*.
11 Lacan, J. (1975–1976). *Le Sinthome*, session of 18.11.75.
12 Lacan, J. (1975–1976). *Le Sinthome*, session of 13.04.76.
13 Lacan, J. (1974–1975). *The Seminar of Jacques Lacan. RSI*. C. Gallagher. (Trans.). Unpublished manuscript, session of 14.01.75. http://www.lacaninireland.com/web/wp-content/uploads/2010/06/RSI-Complete-With-Diagrams.pdf.
14 Lacan, J. (1975–1976). *Le Sinthome*, session of 18.11.75.
15 Lacan, J. (1975–1976). *Le Sinthome*, session of 18.11.75.
16 Allouch, J. (2024). *Where There Is Symptom and Sinthome*.

The intersinthomatic and the plus one of transference

Allouch poses a question to the links that are formed from the transference at the end of an analysis that continues beyond the analysis into the work of a psychoanalytic school. He seems to be pointing to a problem with certain groups which are formed around a social bond where the transferences remain tied with identifications in a closed circuit of the group. I understand that to consider the transferences in a psychoanalytic group or school from the perspective of the intersinthomatic is to consider each transference from its own particular loopings. If we think of the loopings in the Borromean knot whereby if one loop is cut, this frees all the others too, then every transference is singular and particular to each person. I think Allouch's point is that the loops that one's transference effects at the end of an analysis do not just return to the particular manner of the knotting of the symptom which led one to the analysis. Rather, it is a looping that enables something to be worked from the trajectory that one's transference continues to effect. In this way, the intersinthomatic of transference from the end of an analysis does not form a social bond, but it may knock onto other transferences through something that is evoked in the work for each one.

It was precisely to confront the problem of the social bond that organised a group around an identification with an ideal or a master that Lacan proposed the structure of the cartel, and he designated the plus one as a point in the transference that is charged from the work rather than from a point of identification.[17] In the Study Days of the Ecole Freudienne de Paris in April 1975, Lacan nevertheless clarifies that the plus one is always present as not recognised (*méconnu*), and he warns us to take note of this element, which, even if it is not the Other of the Other, can still be incarnated.[18] This incarnation can be in the form of an identification with the father in the symptom or with God as an absolute Other in religion.[19] In his seminar *RSI*, he notes that any social knot is constituted from the hole of the sexual non-rapport, which, even if there are three, makes four.[20] In this context, he considers the plus one from mathematics as +1, which is the additional element, like the number 0, that is at once both outside of the series and counted as part of the series.[21] It seems that this additional +1 element is similar to the fourth loop of the Borromean knot which Lacan later names as the sinthome. As already noted, he considered a sinthome to be this additional loop that was constituted by the way in

17 Lacan, J. (1990 [1964]). *Television: A Challenge to the Psychoanalytic Society*. J Copjec (Ed.), J. Mehlman (Trans.). New York & London: W. W. Norton & Company, p. 97.
18 Journées of the Ecole Freudienne de Paris 12/13 Avril 1975. In: *Lettres de L'Ecole Freudienne de Paris, 18, 1976*. http://www.lacaninireland.com/web/wp-content/uploads/2014/03/Cartel-Study-Days-1975.pdf.
19 Journées of the Ecole Freudienne de Paris 12/13 Avril 1975.
20 Lacan, J. (1974–1975). *The Seminar of Jacques Lacan*, session of 15.04.75.
21 Lacan, J. (1974–1975). *The Seminar of Jacques Lacan*, session of 14.01.75.

which Joyce's writings were enabled by a "charge from the father."[22] We may see this as enabling a writing that continues from a point where the father fails; from beyond the father. I consider that Allouch's concept of the intersinthomatic raises an important point, then, concerning the transference beyond an analysis, and what is enabled of the loops of each transference in the work beyond the limit of the father and a master.

I have often thought about why there has never been a strong value placed on the cartel in the Freudian School of Melbourne, and nevertheless analysts and members in the School continue to write papers which present their work at the yearly Homage conference, as well as in the *Papers of the Freudian School of Melbourne* and in *Écritique*. If the proposition is that the plus one is psychoanalysis, this follows that there is no Other of the Other, and the transmission of psychoanalysis is a work of the transference that continuously confronts the impossible of the traumatising-because-inexistent sexual relation. We can consider the plus one as the intersinthomatic that evokes the additional loop around an Otherness in the transference, around the hole that opens to the real, which challenges each one to continue to write the symbolic in a new way. The papers we have each written from the work of this cartel of translation are produced from our particular transferences to Allouch's paper and to the School. These writings, like ripples in the water that each boat sets in motion, affect the waves of different transferences and charge other writings which produce the psychoanalytic discourse of the Freudian School of Melbourne. This is the necessary of a writing of the impossible of the sexual relation that doesn't stop not being written.

22 Lacan, J. (1975–1976). *The Seminar of Jacques Lacan*, session of 18.11.75.

Chapter 22

Drifting

Megan Williams

I was struck twice during the work that Tine, Michael and I did on the translation of Allouch's paper by the same thought: "I don't know anything about that. I have nothing to say." The first time was when Michael proposed that we speak here about our work of translation. The second time was when Tine raised as a possible discussion point Allouch's linking of sinthome to group, making of it the sinthome of a group. I want to pursue the thoughts that followed my "I know nothing of it and have nothing to say" in each case, and see if they become "something to say."

Regarding translation, the thought that followed was, "Well, we'll talk, and ideas will be discussed, and something will emerge." By this I meant that there is a building or swelling in a working together, even if—or perhaps only if—each person is essentially working alone and following their own current. Others' ideas, as I hear them, send out a small strand or current, sideways, as it were, which I want to follow because it connects to something I have thought, or just affects me. We go away and each work our ideas. Then, when we meet again, the same process occurs. Our work is not the same; the ideas which each of us follows are not the same, even to the extent that it can be surprising to hear one of the others cite something I apparently said in the last meeting, which sent out a strand or a current in their own thoughts, and which I don't recall saying because it wasn't my main current. So each work is different, but when they meet in discussion, something occurs which sends out new currents in again-varied directions. I say this about the meetings of the School as well as the work that we did on the Allouch translation, and I note that Michael has previously proposed that translation is a work of the School, since it's in the School that texts are read and discussed.

I think that this process that I have described may be rhizomatic in the sense developed by Deleuze and Guattari—whose work and commentary on it I have encountered in the seminar of David Pereira, Psychoanalysis, Philosophy and Theology.[1] Rhizomes are extensions of a plant which can make connections from

1 Deleuze, G. and Guattari, F. (2013). *A Thousand Plateaus: Capitalism and Schizophrenia*. London, Oxford, New York, New Delhi, & Sydney: Bloomsbury Academic.

DOI: 10.4324/9781003712480-28

any point along their length to any point on another rhizome. I suppose that, once made, it's impossible, or at least irrelevant, to know which rhizome the connector "belongs" to. Similarly in the School, although each one contributes "my work," what is eventually produced in the meeting cannot be delineated possessively. There is a fruition that comes about in discussions, perhaps especially when we do not understand each other but rather simply take up the thread or current of thought from the other that speaks to us, to me. The different currents at work in and around a discussion swirl apparently chaotically until enough gather in a certain direction to give weight to a swelling that becomes momentarily one thing, a wave—which crests, rides for a while and eventually breaks.

This wave which has become a necessity from the weight of the gathering of small currents isn't really one thing, but for a while, it goes in one direction. It doesn't endure and remain fixed but breaks into many more small currents which shoot off in different directions. After the discussion, different aspects will be taken up by each one and will, in some future gathering, form part of another wave. All waves are different as every gathering is different, even though the settings in which they occur may repeat. Perhaps it is this *gathering together* of the currents into a wave which is what is called the *direction* of the School. What is created—the wave—is beyond every particular one yet is not a knowledge that comes from a big Other in whom we trust. We rather have a certain trust in this process of fruitful gathering of currents within a delimiting that we call psychoanalysis.

Before this starts to sound religious, remember that something, let's say a certain jouissance for each one, is released in the breaking of the wave and then disperses. Perhaps it is wasted—which Lacan says at one point is the only thing you can do with jouissance. Whatever one calls that dispersal, it is a destination for jouissance. In thinking, then, about Tine's remarks about Allouch's idea of a group sinthome (which started a small current in my thoughts), I began to wonder if this forming and breaking of waves is a group sinthome—that process, if I stretch the metaphor to include boats floating on the current, that process which "floats our boats"—though for each one in a different way.

Symptom, and therefore sinthome, are intimately related to jouissance. Lacan speaks of sinthome, I think, as a doing-with jouissance, a knowing-how to do with jouissance. Knowing how to do other than to make a symptom. A *symptom* floats your boat, too, but it's a fixity, a fixed itinerary repeated again and again, the unconscious function of writing the same letter, *encore*, without ceasing. My thought "I don't know anything about that; I have nothing to say" could be called a symptom, or at least the clothing of one. A symptom varies from the process I have been describing in that it is a fixed current always following the same course and also in that it is singular. A symptom does not swell with differences but draws them into its own sameness: a rip rather than a wave. It might need others but takes them as always the same thing: an object or another one of me or the big Other.

A *sinthome*, then, which can meet difference without reducing it to the same, without controlling the process such that the same object of jouissance is always reached, might involve this way of discussing in the School—in which I include the work of translation—that arrives at waves but not final conclusions. Each one might reach a conclusion and take it away to fertilise their next work, but the School itself, in which the waves form and break, made up of all the currents that meet, leaves the questions open: for the next meeting, in which the waves that form have references to the ones that went before but don't conclude them. They are not used for concluding but for fruition, for keeping something going in an indefinitely extended itinerary that no-one knows in advance. And although we make it together, the itinerary and the jouissance of each one is different.

So I come to my other "I don't know," my "I don't have anything to say about translation," of which I will nevertheless say what comes to me, meanderingly, without knowing the itinerary.

One of the words which struck me most in Allouch's paper was his use of the term "beach":

> Lacan [. . .] lodged [the three inexistences] on the same beach as a Borromean knot laid flat, a beach that he claims is that of the "true hole," which is thus not the one where he inscribed the little *a* [. . .]

In our work of translation, we discussed various alternatives to "beach" that might fit better in English with the sense that Allouch seemed to be following. A *jouis-sens*, then, or shared feeling of satisfaction in the current of meaning, of making sense, that gives one (however slightly) the feeling that one knows what he was talking about. In the end, we remained with "beach" because actually, *plage* is a common term that corresponds, as far as one can ever tell what a term from another language corresponds to, to the usage an Anglophone would make of "beach." Why did he use that term? I don't know; I don't really have any sense of the way it is influencing, modifying, the argument he puts; no sense, even, of what effect the word has on me when I read it except a slight discomfort, a rupture or hole in the sense I am making. And yet it evidently has affected me in a way beyond sense and beyond consciousness, since in my writing for today, I have put forward this metaphor of currents and waves breaking on a beach. That is an instance, I think, of what I was trying to speak about earlier: the way in which the work of the School allows that something be channeled and continued but not concluded. "Beach" continued in this one way in my work and will continue in others even though I don't know what Allouch means by it.

There is no apparent hole in sense because one always fills it, but there is a hole in language, an impossibility of pairing, exactly, a word with its partner—a lack of sexual relation and thus an impossibility of translating. One challenge of translating is to allow the hole in language to make a cut in sense; to not close the sense, not form a conclusion which is an occlusion. It may be that keeping open this hole in sense is what allows the other currents to form and take their own direction; that the translation, then, ought to make enough sense that a wave—a working together—can form, but not enough that it never breaks; that it remain a fixity, a common understanding of what is "meant" (recalling here the homophony that Lacan made between "meant" and the French word (*ment*) for lying).

Another term I want to pick out of the many is "adrift." I translated the middle section of the paper, and in doing so, I translated *à la dérive* (p. 5) as "drifting." *A la dérive* is an expression I particularly like. It says to me "with the drift, taken by the current." Allouch writes that the jouissance of the Other, taken as the Othersex, is inexistent yet also *à la dérive*, drifting in the current. It was suggested to me that "adrift" is a better translation than "drifting," and I agreed immediately. "Of course, I thought, that's what one says in English: 'adrift.' Perfect." Yet I realise now that there is some attachment to "drifting." "Drifting" implies to me a choice, while "adrift" suggests a lostness, a shipwreck. "Drifting" touches my jouissance, and it takes the place, fills in for the inexistent jouissance of the Other through the drift of what comes to me from Allouch: fills in for the Other of language, the Other who knows, the big Other of the small other that Allouch is. In the words that I am engaged with, this one resonance affects me in passing, in drifting, *à la dérive*, without me knowing anything of the jouissance of the Othersex, the sex Other than mine. There's no sexual relation because that Other doesn't exist, doesn't enjoy, yet in its place, there is something, the word "drifting," which captivates me and momentarily obscures this hole. Thus saying "Other" can drift, designating in one current an alterity and in another, the place of partner, Other of me.

What I am saying which is relevant to translating, just as to speaking and discussing in the School, is that it is not without involving a certain jouissance. *Jouis-sens* or enjoyment of meaning, certainly, but not only, because of the echoes that the word has beyond meaning. When you read a translation, there is a drifting past of the jouissance of the Othersex, the one other than yours, which doesn't exist yet affects you. It drifts past in the form of echoes that each word has in one's history; in the history of a singular lalangue. It's not an objective process of exchanging one word for another. It's evidently not a sexual relation because that Other who knows, the treasury of signifiers where each one has its pair in each other language, doesn't exist. There's always a signifier missing from the treasury, a hole that you make come into being by seeking that signifier, that one which, by virtue of your search, is missing. But there is also always a way of partially, momentarily making up for the lack of sexual relation: with an object *a* or a *suppléance* found without knowing from the drifting jouissance of the Other insofar as it doesn't exist.

Allouch, as far as I can tell, wants to differentiate between those two ways of dealing with the inexistence of the Other. He puts, I think, the object *a*—let's let the phrase *à la dérive* stand in for it—on the side of the drive, desire and thus the symptom, which obscure or stand in for the inexistence, while a sinthome—the way, perhaps, in which I was unknowingly affected by his word "beach" and then brought that current here to meet your currents to eventually form a wave—holds open the inexistence of the Other and falls on the side of the group. He is interested in practices within a group which can hold open and face the inexistence and not turn it into partner, same, Other of me.

I'm not sure that the object *a* has no place in a sinthome, but I do think that working a translation with others, which we could perhaps call a cartel, can hold open the place of the inexistence of the Other, as can other workings of the School. One's translation is challenged by what others hear or read in a phrase or word, which is different. One is forced to reference other readings, those of psychoanalysis. I don't think there's any right answer to translating, unlike one translator whom I once heard explain the ways in which other translations of Lacan are wrong. He was right but not psychoanalytic. In our work of translation, our discussions referenced psychoanalysis in the different ways that each of us had encountered it during our long trajectories with it. There were references to people in Denmark, to English with a capital E, to readings of Lacan that had occurred over many years and to the School and the history of usages in the School. These are currents. Their meeting did not make them the same or produce a fixed agreement, but they produced a wave: this translation of Allouch's paper which we present to the School. That is why, taking up Allouch's proposal, I think that the work of the School can at times function as sinthome, as a making present of the inexistence of the Other in a way which allows a drifting of the jouissance without knowing anything about it, such that the different speakings come together to make a few waves rather than a symptom. It's not a knowing but a *savoir faire*, a knowing how to do with.

Chapter 23

There is no sexual relation, and the social bond

Michael Gerard Plastow

What is translation? As I have cited elsewhere, a primer of French English translation states from the outset that, "Translation is concerned with meaning."[1] Whilst that might be the case for technical translations and may also be part of what is required for any translation, it can never be an adequate definition for a psychoanalytic translation. A recently published book of the translations of the three major papers that I studied in my book on the writings of Sabina Spielrein begins in the following way: "translating Spielrein's medical dissertation into *readable* English was a daunting task."[23] Other translations promote notions of a 'faithful' translation. These notions of readability and faithfulness themselves promote a priori notions of the function and method of translations.

By contrast, Walter Benjamin, in his essay *The Task of the Translator*, proposes that "a translation [. . .] must lovingly and in detail incorporate the original's mode of signification."[4] Here, there is love involved, and this love is our transference-love to our work of translation in reference to The Freudian School of Melbourne. And if there is love, there is certainly also jouissance—mostly experienced as suffering, *souffrance*—which might be heard in French as *sous France*, or 'under France,' perhaps here under the yoke of the French language—in the translation from that language. When Freud cites *traduttore traditore*, or 'translator traitor,' there is a betrayal in the translation; however, the work of translation also betrays something of this suffering, or jouissance, of the translator. And part of our suffering in translation is due to the fact that between languages, *there is no sexual relation*: There is no ratio or correspondence or equivalence between French and

1 Hervey, S. and Higgins, I. (2002). *Thinking French Translation*. London: Routledge, p. 132.
2 Plastow, M. G. (2019). *Sabina Spielrein and the Poetry of Psychoanalysis: Writing and the End of Analysis*. London: Routledge.
3 Cape, R. I. and Burt, R. (2019). *The Essential Writings of Sabina Spielrein*. London: Routledge, p. ix, (my italics).
4 Benjamin, W. (1999). The task of the translator. In: *Illuminations*. London: Pimlico, p. 79.

DOI: 10.4324/9781003712480-29

English. To propose a definitive translation is to invoke a definitive failure. Jorge Luis Borges proposed the following:

> Bilingual dictionaries [. . .] make us believe that each word of a language can be replaced by another from another language. The error consists in not taking into account that each language is a mode of experiencing and perceiving the universe.[5]

I have long thought that psychoanalytic translation could be approximated to the translation of poetry. This was one of the reasons I was keen to have the seminar of Lacan's that I translated published in a bilingual edition just as poetry is often published. In this way, the translation is never definitive, nor does it have to be slavishly faithful or fear betrayal, since it is always referred to the original text.[6] If poetry were translated just for meaning, it would be a very ordinary translation. If one translates for meaning, it implies that one knows, or is able to decide, what the meaning is. In psychoanalysis, however, we must allow for the play of the signifier in order to not foreclose on meaning lest we reduce what is translated to merely 'readable' English. We must, wherever possible, allow the signifiers and the structure of the other language—French in this case—to pass into English. Where this is not possible, we need to find words that again do not foreclose on meaning. In any case, it is rare that a word has just one meaning. One word has a whole scope or range of meanings—amply demonstrated by consulting a dictionary regarding the word *plage* from this paper of Allouch in French, in which the entries indicate the literal meaning of 'beach,' plus all the figurative significations that follow from the function of a beach such as a border, a field or area, an intermediate zone that separates land from sea, etc., etc., for which we have to then find a term in English that approximates such a scope, or significations, or to translate it literally as we have chosen to do here.[7]

Any translation is nonetheless ultimately a type of interpretation, but the interpretation could be just a conventional interpretation into meaning. Here, the effort is to transmit the elements of the text and to allow them to retain their structure and their mode of relation to each other—that is, their mode of signification—we could say their topological relation. This question pertains to our choice of English words in the translation. This was part of our task in the final stage of bringing the three parts of the translation together so that we can track the progress of the signifier by a particular word being translated by the same word in English in a different place

5 Cited in: Rodríguez Ponte, R. E. (November 1986). Traducción y Traducción. In: *Notas de la Escuela Freudiana*, no. 5, Escuela Freudiana de Buenos Aires, p. 25.

6 Lacan, J. (2013). *Le Savoir du Psychanalyste/The Knowledge of the Psychoanalyst: Séminaire 1971–1972* (Bilingual edition). M. Plastow (Trans.). Paris: Éditions de l'Association Lacanienne Internationale. (Non-commercial edition).

7 Rey, A. (2013). *Le Grand Robert* (Dictionnaire Électronique). Paris: Le Robert.

in the text or at least indicating a change of choice of term. As Allouch writes in this text in regard to the symptom and sinthome:

> [T]hey are composed of statements and mathemes, which can vary and which can therefore only be read [or translated, we could add] by considering their progressions, their variations, and their transformations. Varity [*Varité*], better than truth [*vérité*].

And Lacan put forward in the seminar The Knowledge of the Psychoanalyst that "In psychoanalysis, the symptom has to do with something that is the translation into words of its value of truth."[8] So writing, and translating, also concerns the value of truth, or even the varity of verity. And writing is also concerned with knowing what to do with the symptom and, we can add, with one's sinthome.

Together, we spoke about how difficult it was to speak about Allouch's paper without being influenced by it. I found myself thinking in this reductive sort of way: Is this "the analytics of the object a" or that of "there is no sexual relation"? For this reason, I find it necessary to try to say something now of what Allouch proposes of this analytics of "there is no sexual relation" *and* the sinthome of the group.

Sinthome of the group

Given that I initially translated the latter third of the paper, I wrestled with the translation of this term "*sinthome de groupe*." It could be rendered as "group sinthome," but that would give it a possessive sense in English, implying that the sinthome in this case is that of the group. But can there be a sinthome that encompasses more than one subject? This led me to consider that it is better translated as "sinthome of the group," which would allow the equivocation of both the "group's sinthome" as well as the "sinthome's group," the group that pertains to—or rather is defined by—the sinthome. In any case, I found this group sinthome rather puzzling, in particular because of this word "group," which evokes a group psychology. It becomes clear that what Allouch is referring to is a 'psychoanalytic group,' which is effectively an oxymoron. In our context, we would have to consider this to be a "sinthome of the School," a school then which is no longer a group.

The sinthome is no doubt fabricated by an art or an artifice, or a savoir-faire, and Allouch indicates that the analyst provisionally incarnates the sinthome, at least the sinthome of the analysand. So if the sinthome is fabricated in the analysis, then it can be deployed by the analyst in the psychoanalytic school. So then the *sinthome de groupe* is not so much the group's sinthome but rather the sinthome's group—thus for the sinthome of the School—a school in which the sinthome can be put to work.

8 Lacan, J. (1971–1972). *The Seminar of Jacques Lacan Book XIX*, p. 59.

However, the other difficulty to consider is the question of what sort of group or school is specified by the sinthome, whose "analytics" are determined by a negative statement: There is no sexual relation. Megan put forward: "I don't know anything about it." Thus there is no sexual relation, and there is no knowledge. And by a certain looseness of usage, one often hears some refer to 'the no sexual relation' or 'the non-sexual relation,' as if this were some positivised entity, like a particular mode of relation that could be specified. This would be to substantialise what is not substantial.

Even though Allouch does not clarify how this might function, he writes about the transferences of an intersinthomatic order—which is a tautology, since he has already defined the intersinthomatic relations as transference. Nonetheless, here, the un-looped transferences refer to transferences that are active but not fixed: "suspended," he also writes. In other words, this is a transference that is carried beyond one's individual analysis and is available for work within the psychoanalytic school. For our ad hoc cartel of translation, the plus one is designated as the School, since the translation is done specifically in reference to the School—and in the first instance only circulated within the School—making it apt that we first presented it at the Seminar of the Freudian School of Melbourne.

Since this group sinthome is underwritten by the declaration that "there is no sexual relation," and it is the different modalities of the sexual relation that determine the social bond, we must conclude that the sinthome of the group does not determine any social bond whatsoever in regard to a psychoanalytic school. If it did, then it would indeed make of the school a group. And of course, each psychoanalytic school risks reducing itself to a group and to functioning as a group the more it emphasises a social bond that unifies and provides an identifying rod—a lightning rod for identifications—and the more the plus one is embodied, or incorporated, in one or more people.

On the contrary, analysis can only serve to loosen such bonds or to dissolve them, such that the transference may be put to work in the School. Or to put this in another way, if we examine the four discourses, the top line of each discourse defines each of the particular modalities of the social bond in so far as the agent addresses the other. As Lacan said, "There results from this that I have defined certain types of 'discourses,' as being what establishes a defined type of social bond."[9] So in the upper line of the discourse of the hysteric, the divided subject addresses the master, or master signifier; in the discourse of the analyst, the analyst in the place of the semblant of the object a is faced with the divided subject and so on. Each of these forms of sexual relation—or social bond—however, is marked by its own impossibility, an impossibility that leads on, in the lower line of the discourses, to the impotence of each of the discourses, promoting a change of discourse. This impossibility is effectively the impossibility of the social bond

9 Lacan, J. (1971–1972). *Ou pire: Séminaire 1971–1972*. Paris: Éditions de l'Association Lacanienne Internationale, 2008, p. 47. (Non-commercial edition).

of a psychoanalytic school. This is not to say that such social bonds do not exist but that they are incompatible with the functioning of a psychoanalytic school. So, in so far as the sinthome of the group is determined by "there is no sexual relation," it is only determined by the discourses and the social bond by virtue of the very impossibility of this sexual relation and therefore the instability of the social bond.

We can conclude from this that the sinthome of the group does not form any social bond of its own. Of course, it does not stop social bonds from being operative and from being symptomatic in a school's functioning. But it is rather a question of what to do with the symptom for it to function as sinthome. Whilst one is at once inspired and enthused by the others with whom one works to produce something, a work that is properly psychoanalytic is nonetheless only produced outside of the sexual relation. Thus it is outside of the love and hate and ignorance of the passions of being, outside even of the friendships, the collegiality and the camaraderie with one's colleagues. And it is to be noted that even though the members of a cartel work together, they sustain a reference point outside the cartel—here a plus one embodied by the Freudian School of Melbourne. And it is thus that each can produce something not as a joint work but something singular produced each in his or her own name.

Part VII

Melbourne Seminars of Christian Fierens 2019

Chapter 24

Introduction to four seminars by Christian Fierens

Debbie Plastow, Editor of the Fierens papers

Christian Fierens is a psychoanalyst practising in Tervuren, near Brussels, as well as a prodigious author, publishing innumerable books and articles on psychoanalysis, including interrogation of the works of Freud and Lacan. Fierens is not one to be deterred by obscurities and enigmas in the seminars and writings of Lacan, as evident from his earliest publications, such as *Lecture de L'Etourdit* (l'Hermattan, 2002), translated in English as *Reading L'Etourdit.*

In 2015, Fierens was first invited to present a series of seminars at the Freudian School of Melbourne, including presenting at the Homage to Lacan, held in the University of Melbourne's 1888 Building. These seminars were later edited and published in Volume 26 of the *Papers of the Freudian School of Melbourne*, *Lacan and Other Heresies: Lacanian Psychoanalytic Writings.*

Fierens was invited to present a second series of seminars in Melbourne in August 2019. The four papers included in the current volume were written specifically by Fierens for these public lectures, held at Australian Catholic University in Fitzroy. He later agreed for the seminars to be edited for publication in the *Papers of the Freudian School of Melbourne*. The changes made aimed to increase readability, for the papers to 'sound more English,' but without losing the sense of Otherness, inherent in the style and cadence of Fierens' speech. Additionally, it was necessary to retain particular signifiers that insisted through his presentations. When asked whether he had original versions in French, Fierens replied, "I don't have a French version. I always try to write directly in English to keep in touch with the audience."

Keeping in touch with the audience was precisely what Christian Fierens achieved during his two visits to Melbourne. Despite a busy schedule of seminars, he generously presented lectures and provided supervision to different audiences, including Alfred Child and Youth Mental Health Services (CYMHS), Austin CYMHS, and SPECTRUM, as well as meeting individually with School members, exemplifying his dedication to the work of psychoanalysis. He also launched the English translation of his book *The Soul of Narcissism* (Routledge, 2019) at Readings in Carlton.

On being asked about his quotations and reference sources, Fierens explained that he had used few direct quotations from texts and did not have many references

DOI: 10.4324/9781003712480-31

in English, adding, "There are also fictitious quotations from people I let speak." In this statement, we can hear that although his presentations are underpinned by extensive reading and interrogation of the texts of Freud, Lacan, Kant and others, Fierens places emphasis on listening to and reflecting on the words of those he allows to speak, from the couch.

Fierens' insistence on letting people speak, without judgement, was evident when he first presented at the Freudian School of Melbourne's 2015 *Homage to Lacan*. When a participant previously unknown to the School presented himself to the audience, I was moved by Fierens' attentive listening and humble, considered responses, which provoked lively discussion and set the tone for the rest of the conference.

There are four papers in this volume. In his first paper, "Reality and Truth," Fierens begins with a questioning, not only asking his listener, "What does this mean?" and "What is to be done?" but "*How* can it be done?" In this and each of the subsequent papers, Fierens explores and interrogates Kant's *Critique of Pure Reason*, a work comprising a prelude to his book, *Tenir pour Vrai* (Hermann, 2020). Fierens explains that the Kantian expression, holding as true—*Für Wahr halten*—entails three manners of approaching truth, namely, knowledge, faith and opinion. In his book, Fierens proposes an additional approach to holding as true: repression.

In "Sexuality and Narcissism," Fierens states at the outset: "I do not require the title of analyst in order to begin to speak as an analyst, and then to hold my discourse as the discourse of an analyst." In an exploration of transference and identification via the four discourses, he concludes that "the end of analysis is not the identification of the analysand" but, rather, the practice of psychoanalysis "awakens and sparks the movement of the unconscious."

"Symptom and Sinthome" provokes a questioning of the notion of the unconscious. Beginning with Freud's statement, "It does not think, calculate or judge in any way at all," Fierens asks, "*How* does the unconscious work?" and answers, "It invents a new form." He then extends his question into the clinic, asking, "What does this mean for our practice?"

"Enjoyment and Sexual Disorientation" continues to explore and to question the work of Lacan and Kant, specifically in relation to Kant's moral law, extending this theorisation to notions of the unconscious, the original sin, sexuality, and his invention of the jouissance principle. As always, this is related to the clinic and the place of the analyst, who must begin with failure and invent something new.

Fierens' presentations and presence at public lectures and the Homage of the Freudian School of Melbourne have created the momentum for us to invent something new. By letting him speak, we have an opportunity to engage in ideas from outside of the School. This dedication to psychoanalysis, evidenced also in Fierens' wealth of papers and texts, propels us to pursue such a work.

Chapter 25

Reality and truth

Christian Fierens

Science acts as if it had the reality of its objects in front of it, "existing" independently of its discourse. The common man thinks that there is a reality of different kinds of objects—food, clothes, tools, instruments, houses, cars, and perhaps even wife, husband and children—independently of his discourse.

This can work rather well. Generally, science obtains good results. Science can predict a lot of things and allows the common man to deal with the objects of his daily life. He acts as though the reality of his objects existed prior to his research and his desire. But this is not true. His object is always constructed in the framework of the questions of scientific research or in the framework of questions, desires and interests of the common man. Pure reality is not true, but it works. Thus, we don't have a complete truth that would tally with reality. We have just the half-said of truth when it works.

It would be simple and comfortable if the psychologist, the psychiatrist or the psychoanalyst could do the same as science and the common man with a half-truth. By believing in this reality, and more specifically, in the reality of mental diseases, the practitioner could build up a lot of theoretical and practical results. He would be able to get to the point all the more quickly if he were able to think in the same way as the common man who consults him. But this is not true. Perhaps it is half-true. So where is this half-truth?

Every psychopathological problem—neurosis, psychosis, and so on—is dependent upon the discourse in which it arose. But there is more than that. The symptom, which is always presented in the framework of discourse and of transference, remains essentially a fact of discourse that is impossible to reduce to a realistic fact or a realistic object. Of course, the psychiatrist can take up a scientific position, but then the genuine psychical symptom has disappeared to make room for a bunch of data to be treated with statistics. Is this reality? This will depend upon the position of the psychiatrist, his statistics and his discourse, and changes according to the fluctuations of the psychiatrist and of the edition of his diagnostic and statistical manual. There is no genuine reality of psychopathology. It is a fiction. It is created by discourse.

The first and foremost prerequisite for psychoanalysis is to rid itself of the realism of science and of the common man to enter the world of discourse. Henceforth

DOI: 10.4324/9781003712480-32

we have to consider how psychological things are done just with the saying. For my first talk four years ago, I chose a title in accordance with Austin's title, "How to do things with words."[1] These are performative utterances. For example, if the judge says to the accused, "I condemn you to five years in prison," he is convicted in so far as this magistrate is empowered to do such a thing. The same applies to a wedding, a bequest, and so on. You say it and it is done, whatever your intention may be.

Can we say that doing with the saying in the psychological field is the same as the aforementioned performative utterances? Not at all. Here we cannot find the magistrate who is empowered to do such things with words. Or would you say 'the unconscious'? But the unconscious ". . . does not think, calculate or judge in any way at all; it restricts itself to giving things a new form."[2] There is no magistrate in the unconscious. The saying-doing in our psychoanalytic field is quite different from the simple saying-doing of performative utterances, but it is also more general.

If the unconscious does not end up in performative utterances, where does this lead? It seems doomed to err in countless repetitions, unsolvable contradictions, aimless drives, and foolish transferences. These are the four fundamental concepts of psychoanalysis. Nonetheless, they seem to go nowhere at all. It is time to take stock of these wanderings. Psychoanalytic interpretation cannot do better than providing equivocal interpretations that never arrive at fact or reality. Even Lacan's *object a* as unrepresentable remains a process of questioning: is it something or is it nothing?

With such lack of reality, we are far from truth. We do not have any truth at all. As everything is a fiction, every apparent certitude is suspected of being phoney, a sham, bogus, and the psychoanalytic discourse mere humbug. Nevertheless, we are claiming that psychoanalysis is a practice of truth, from truth and for truth. What does this mean? What is truth?

In his essay, "On the Essence of Truth" (1943),[3] Heidegger poses a question regarding truth as independent of any practical experience, technical consideration, scientific research, even thoughtful reflection or religion. He asks, "Yet with this question concerning essence do we not soar too high into the void of generality which deprives all thinking of breath?"[4]

A true object	A true sentence

1 Austin, J. L. (1962). *How to Do Things with Words: The William James Lectures Delivered at Harvard University in 1955*. J. O. Urmson and M. Sbisà (Eds.). Oxford: Clarendon Press.

2 Freud, S. (1900a). The interpretation of dreams. SE IV-V: 507.

3 https://media.aphelis.net/wp-content/uploads/2011/02/Martin-Heidegger-On-the-Essence-of-Truth.pdf

4 https://media.aphelis.net/wp-content/uploads/2011/02/Martin-Heidegger-On-the-Essence-of-Truth.pdf, p. 1.

For us, it is impossible to avoid the question of the essence of truth, because we are confronted with a world of semblances. Moreover, we aim to find the truth of the unconscious. Here we can speak of a true object or of a true sentence. In both instances it is an agreement.

A true object: For example, we speak of 'true gold' in distinction from false. False gold is not actually what it appears to be. It is merely a 'semblance.' Genuine or true gold is in agreement with what, always and in advance, we 'properly' mean by 'gold.' To be true is to be in agreement. *Das stimmt*. Truth is agreement. True gold was the reference standard for all monetary and commercial transactions across the globe. As such, it appeared to be a true reality, independent of everything else. It was able to be unconditionally trusted. Do we have such a true object, a standard reference, in the psychoanalytic field?

For Freud, the reference standard is surely the phallus. But the phallus is not an object. It is, rather, a process that is endlessly relaunching psychical movement. It is not possible to find an agreement in the phallic function. An exception outside of the phallic function that arranged everything in the phallic field does not exist. *Das stimmt nicht*. It is not in agreement.

For Lacan, the reference standard would be the object *a*. However, although the object *a* seems to be an object, it is not a real object that is in agreement with what we mean here. In the gap between something and nothing, it is impossible to represent it without losing its most important part: the question of nothing. *Das stimmt nicht*. The psychoanalytic reference standard disappears. It seems impossible to find a true object. The question of truth and of its agreement remains.

A true sentence: A proposition is true if what it says is in accordance with the object about which the statement is made. It is in agreement. *Das stimmt*.

Do we have true sentences in the psychoanalytic field? True interpretations? For Freud, it is impossible to find the umbilicus of the dream. We always miss the point. And for Lacan, the interpretation must always remain equivocal. Complete agreement is never reached. We do not have a single true sentence in psychoanalysis. The question of truth and of its agreement remains. When we speak of a true object or of a true sentence, we always mean an agreement. The object must be in agreement with the sentence which describes the genuine object. The sentence must be in agreement with the object which is spoken about. *Adaequatio rei ad intellectum and adaequatio intellectus ad rem*.

Now we must discuss the concept of *adaequatio*—agreement—all the more so since psychoanalysis typically emphasises discordance, conflict, and disharmony. How is it possible to find an accordance or a correspondence between two such diverse things as an object and a sentence? Any correspondence is only possible on the grounds of an open stance that entails objects and sentences in the questioning of Dasein. It is only on the grounds of the inner possibility of a being-in-the-world that the correctness of the sentence, or proposition, gives the appearance of fulfilling the essence of truth. Open stance in regard to all beings means "to let beings be the beings they are." This sounds a little abstract or repetitive. But it is quite concrete. We try to attain this every day in the practice of free association: let beings be what they are, let sayings be. Heidegger calls this 'freedom.'

Freedom is openness to everything in the world of saying. The essence of truth is no longer agreement, but what makes this agreement possible. And this is freedom. The essence of truth is freedom. Freedom is not at all the capacity to do everything. It is an openness to every side of every being.

Letting beings be, which is an attuning, a bringing into accord, prevails throughout and anticipates all the open comportment that flourishes in it. 'Truth' in Greek is *alètheia* which means 'disclosure,' 'unclosedness,' 'unconcealedness.' But depending on the aforesaid freedom, truth, *alètheia*, also entails concealment. We know this perfectly well in psychoanalysis: "nothing is hidden so much as what is unveiled, as truth, *Alètheia* = *Verborgenheit*."[5] When we think that we have a good interpretation, unveiling the unconscious, we soon discover that it is only a screen interpretation or a screen memory. With freedom, as the essence of truth, we know that not wanting to know, or concealment, is an integral part of truth. It is not an accident in the field of truth. Heidegger mentions that concealment, which appears as untruth, points to the still unexperienced domain of the truth of Being (Sein), not merely of beings.

Henceforth, taking the essence of truth into account is taking into account the fact that man errs, not just waiting to find the end of his errancy and the revelation of truth. He is always astray in errancy, because as ek-sistent he in-sists and so is already caught in errancy. So, we know that truth is not a point or a stance. It is a movement. What can we do with this truth? What must we do if we wish to remain in the movement of truth, in its pathway, which is in its method? How can we deal with this truth which is always escaping?

We never possess truth. At the beginning of *Television*, Lacan says: "I always speak the truth. Not the whole truth, because there's no way, to say it all. Saying it all is literally impossible: words fail. Yet it's through this very impossibility that the truth holds onto the real."[6] Is he not bragging when he says he always speaks the truth? He? Who? It is not only Lacan who always speaks the truth. It is every analysand, every speaker, because concealment and lying are no more than standpoints within the essence of truth and its openness, in freedom. And the analyst must take charge of this fact, which is truth in the saying of the analysand.

Truth is neither the whole truth nor one truth. For example, when somebody is consciously lying, saying a falsehood, surely, he does not hold it as true, yet he holds it as true in so far as he wants you to believe it. And by doing so, he has the true purpose of cheating you concerning the object or the fact that he is talking

5 Lacan, J. (1972). L'Étourdit. C. Gallagher (Trans.). In: *The Letter: 41*, Summer 2009.

6 Lacan, J. (1987 [1973]). *Television*. D. Hollier, R. Krauss and A. Michelson (Trans.). *October: 40*. Cambridge, MA & London: MIT, p. 7.

about. Hence, we have a very complex set of figures of holding as true, depending on what is held as true (the object considered in the process of truth) and on who is holding it as true (the subject committed in the process of truth).

Depending on the object	Depending on the subject

More precisely, this depends on the place and the function of the so-called object and on the place and the function of the so-called subject.

Saint Augustine advised distinguishing *intelligere*, to understand or to know, *credere*, to believe, and *opinari*, to have a mere opinion.[7] We owe what we know to reason or to the objectivity of the object. We owe what we believe to our subjectivity depending on the authority of God, for example.

To know the object	The belief of the subject

But what about when reason fails? Whoever has opinions claims to know what he does not know. To know, to believe and to have opinions are three quite different types of holding something as true. With these three kinds of holding as true, we are no longer focused on the difference between 'true' or 'false,' but on the reasons for holding as true. Is it possible to find them in the object? Then we have knowledge. Is it possible to find these reasons in the subject? Then we have belief. Or are there no sufficient reasons at all to hold as true? Then we have mere opinion.

As we never have truth, we seek it and we always speak the truth by means of holding as true. And these means are dependent on the object and the subject, and on their relations. In the methodology of his *Critique of Pure Reason*, Kant distinguishes three kinds of holding as true (*Fürwahrhalten*), according to the sufficiency and insufficiency of different kinds of reasons for holding as true. When the objective and subjective reasons are sufficient, we have some knowledge (*Wissen*). When the objective reasons are insufficient but the subjective one is sufficient, we have some faith or belief (*Glauben*). When the objective and subjective reasons are insufficient, we have opinion (*Meinen*).

	Objectively sufficient	*Objectively not sufficient*
Subjectively sufficient	Knowledge	Faith or belief
Subjectively not sufficient	???	Opinion

7 Saint Augustine, *De utilitate credendi*, XI 25, quoted by Jacques Lebrun: "Vérité scientifique et vérité historique à l'âge classique." In Lebrun, J. (2007). *La vérité, entre psychanalyse et philosophie*. M. Plon and H. Rev-Flaud (Dir.). Toulouse: érès.

It seems that Kant does no more than remind us of Saint Augustine's trilogy. Yet, with Kant, the sufficiency of the subjective reason is not the authority of God—of a big Other—as was the case with Saint Augustine, but it is the authority or the autonomy of practical reason (which entails freedom). What does this mean for us? Where is our practical reason? Not in God, nor in Freud or Lacan. When we are practising psychoanalysis, lacking any kind of big Other, who guarantees our practice? We do not have sufficient objective reasons to hold the unconscious as true: objectively, it is not conscious. So, it is impossible to have genuine knowledge of the unconscious. However, when we want to practise psychoanalysis, in our practice and for our practice, we have sufficient subjective reason to hold it as true. We believe in it and so we can begin with free associations, and so on.

When we are looking at the structure of these manners of holding as true, an oddity or an anomaly is striking. In order to distribute these modalities, there are two criteria: are the reasons sufficient or not? Does it come from the object or from the subject? So, we would expect four manners of holding as true: a reason objectively and subjectively sufficient, and that is knowledge; a reason objectively insufficient and subjectively sufficient, and that is belief or faith; a reason objectively and objectively insufficient, and that is opinion. But in the previous schema we have an empty box. Obviously the fourth one—a reason objectively sufficient and subjectively insufficient—is lacking, for Kant as well as for Saint Augustine. It was impossible for them to imagine that a sane subject would decline to accept objective pieces of evidence.

Nevertheless, in the psychoanalytic field, this place—the empty box—is quite conspicuous. In regard to the most important aspects of his life, the analysand does not want to know. That is, we have certitude of some objective facts and he does not give his subjective approval. The subjective reason for holding it as true is lacking. This holding as true, when the objective evidence does not reach the subjective approbation, is at stake in neurosis as 'repression' (*Verdrängung*), in psychosis as 'foreclosure' (*Verwerfung*) and in perversion as 'disavowal' (*Verleugnung*). For each of these types of psychopathology, we will keep in mind the general form of declining to give his subjective assent to a fact or a thing that is objective. There the objective reason is sufficient, but subjectively, it is quite insufficient. This is repression in the general meaning of the word.

For Kant and other philosophers, this was inconceivable. If you did not accept objective reason, you could be accused of bad faith (not of repression), and they rendered it as the second holding as true, to faith, but a bad one. Nowadays, we have to cope with four manners of holding as true. Here is the table of the different modalities:

	Objectively sufficient	*Objectively insufficient*
Subjectively sufficient	Knowledge	Faith or belief
Subjectively insufficient	Repression	Opinion

With knowledge, we have sufficient objective reasons for holding as true: the object is taken as a sufficiently reliable reality. Moreover, the subjective reasons are also sufficient in so far as the subject is conceived of as having the same mechanics as the object. The questioning inherent to the subject has disappeared completely or it is just a matter of God. So the very question of the subject is always already more or less repressed in knowledge. That is the genuine holding as true of science, which in fact does not take into account the subjectivity of the researcher or of God.

With repression—sufficient objective reasons, but insufficient subjectively—the questioning of the subject comes back: the return or the breakthrough of the repressed. And with it, the questioning of the object takes another turn. What is an object if its so-called reality is not compelling us towards truth? Repression—which appears as an "I do not want to know, I do not want to be clammed up in knowledge"—appears then as the questioning of the object as such: "Is it something to be really trusted or nothing?" Repression entails this question, that is, it entails Lacan's object *a*.

With faith—no sufficient objective reason, but sufficient subjective reasons—the questioning of the object is put aside, in relation to knowledge as well as to repression. The subject appears to be sufficient to its holding as true. But this subject is not to be seen as a so-called individual or object, but as the result, the effect, of a practice, of a process, for example, the process of the unconscious. So, the subject is not a common subject at all. The latter must be barred in order to make way for the practice that entails the subject as an effect.

With opinion—no sufficient reasons either subjective nor objective—each 'said' is put on the same level as another. Its meaning has no importance, except that with these 'saids' you begin to speak and imagine knowledge, repress this knowledge, and begin to believe in the process. Everything can begin with a mere opinion of no importance, no importance except that it unfolds the process of holding as true.

In psychoanalysis, as is the case everywhere, we are prone to search for knowledge. If we were conscious of everything, all would go well, everything would be okay and everybody happy. The psychoanalytic process is seen as a process towards the knowledge of the unconscious and towards the arrangement of everything. And we have tools to reach it. For example, when a patient says that this person in his dream is not his mother, we well know that this is a negation. So it is quite easy, we know that this person is actually his mother. But with such 'knowledge,' nothing is changed, nothing is moved. Anticipating knowledge is surely not the pathway for psychoanalysis. Because knowledge is not truth, it is only one modality, and not the best one, of holding as true. It is surely a wrong one when it takes the central place in regard to truth.

We must move then between the four modalities of holding as true and we must alternately promote each of them, instead of solely focusing on knowledge. Giving way to truth through holding as true always occurs in discourse. Here we do not consider discourse from the point of view of its semblance, or semblant, but from the point of view of its truth, that is, of the unconscious reasons that are at stake in it.

When promoting opinion as true, we are taking any signifier as a mere possibility of truth, without sufficient reasons; we are building up a discourse which seems to be a discourse of knowledge. But it is only a semblance—or a semblant. This is called the academic discourse.

Semblance:	Other:
Academic knowledge	Object *a*
Truth:	Product:
Opinion	Subject

When promoting faith as true, we are taking the question of the subject—not the subject as an individual—as holding as true. We are led by a watchword, an instruction, a call, a master signifier which seems to command discourse. But these are mere semblances. We name this the discourse of the master. But as a matter of fact, it is the discourse of faith, of belief.

Semblance:	Other:
Master signifier	Knowledge
Truth:	Product:
Faith or belief	Object a

When we promote repression as true, we are in the discourse of the hysteric. It seems that it is the hysteric who is provoking a turmoil. But this is only a semblance, because the so-called hysteric is moved by the question of the *object a* and its repression.

Semblance:	Other:
Hysteric subject	Signifier
Truth:	Product
Repression of object a	Knowledge

When we promote knowledge as true, it appears that we are in the scientific discourse or the academic discourse. But we do not have truth. Truly, we do not know what the object is, nor do we know the subject. The truth of knowledge is that we have to question the object and the subject, starting with the object, that is, the object *a*.

Semblance:	Other:
Psychoanalytic object a	Subject
Truth:	Product:
Knowledge	Signifier

Starting from the essence of truth, these discourses are no longer named by their semblance, but by their holding as true. This creates two major differences. Firstly, we no longer think that the semblance is holding its discourse, but that the semblance is held by its truth, the process in freedom of truth. It is discourse which is producing the semblance, and not the contrary.

Secondly, with the nomination of the discourses by their semblance, it seemed that we had a fixed point, the reality of the semblance which is not moving, and so we were established for a long time in a specific discourse. With the nomination of the discourses by their holding as true, we know that truth is always escaping and that we must provisionally hold something. We are always moving between the four discourses.

In dealing with the discourses, taking into account the holding as true instead of the semblance completely changes psychoanalytic practice. The primary aim of Freudian psychoanalytic process was to know the unconscious and to also let the patient know it. From the beginning until the end of the treatment, everything was focused on this knowledge which would allow the identity and the symptoms of the individual to be fixed. However, we know perfectly well that such knowledge does not effect much change in his symptoms.

Now, with truth as freedom, we must equally take into account each of the four manners of holding as true. Let us return to the old example: "This person in my dream is not my mother." This seems to be a knowledge that the analysand communicates to the analyst. In face of this, the analyst knows that it *is* actually his mother. Here two kinds of knowledge are opposed. Who is right? And who is wrong? As long as the analyst remains in the framework of knowledge and tries to convince the patient of his knowledge as truth, he cannot take stock of the other holdings as true that are at stake in this instance.

First of all, we must consider repression. The analysand does not wish to know about his mother. Maybe he does not want his mother to know about him. Surely refusing the fact of his mother could be diagnosed as a discourse of the hysteric. However, he does not wish to be clammed up in the field of his mother who wanted to know him perfectly. Furthermore, perhaps he does not want to be trapped in what the analyst could know about him and without him. Anyway, repression has its grounds, and these are probably more important than to know the possible identity of this person and of his dreams.

Secondly, starting from his subjective position, namely having taken stock of repression, he really believes that it is not his mother and with this master discourse position, he has built his way of life, perhaps a neurotic one. But we do not need to erase his faith. On the contrary, his belief can be the grounds upon which to build a new life. With his mother no longer in position of big Other, he will no longer be trapped into believing in God or in mother. He has to believe now in himself, and more precisely, in the unconscious forces which are engaged in his fight with his mother.

Thirdly, "it is his mother;" "it is not his mother;" "he believes in God;" "he does not believe." Each of these statements alone is objectively and subjectively insufficient. Each is mere opinion. But each of these statements has its place in the roundabout of the process of holding as true.

Fourthly, this roundabout exists as the questioning of the essence of the object and of the subject. But then, knowledge has become something quite other than science. It is the knowledge that we never have the given reality of an object or a subject. "What the analyst must know is how to ignore what he knows." "Ignoring what he knows" means entering into the roundabout of the four manners of holding as true or into the roundabout of the four discourses. There is reality as given. Truth—freedom—is only attainable in the movement of this roundabout.

A psychoanalytic interpretation is not a statement. It is not the communication of a knowledge. It is not the communication of a belief. It is not the consequence of a repression. It is not a mere opinion. Each genuine interpretation is a movement in which holding as true is continually changing. This is the aim of the equivocal side of interpretation. When the interpretation follows this pathway, in relation to, for example, "this person is not my mother," the analysand begins to completely change his manner of being in the world. His world is no longer encompassed in a motherly one. His world has changed completely and with it, his relation to freedom and truth.

Chapter 26

Sexuality and narcissism

Christian Fierens

We are caught up in the field of truth and its freedom. But we never possess truth. The only possibility is holding as true, sometimes as knowledge, sometimes as faith, sometimes as repression, sometimes as opinion. We are caught up in at least one of these four discourses that are not truth, but holding as true.[1]

Knowledge	Faith (belief)
Discourse of the analyst?	Discourse of the master?
Repression	Opinion
Discourse of the hysteric?	Discourse of the academic?

We immediately imagine that we are acting in this discourse, but this is not the case. For example, I do not require the title of analyst in order to begin to speak as an analyst, and then to hold my discourse as the discourse of an analyst. On the contrary, psychoanalytic discourse is working incidentally, and then it sometimes happens that there is a point that seems to function as the agent of psychoanalytic discourse. Nevertheless, we are obsessed by what seems to be the agent of discourse. We imagine the starting point of each discourse: the discourse of faith would begin with a master, the discourse of repression would begin with a hysteric, the discourse of opinion would begin with an academic, and the discourse of knowledge would begin with an analyst who is supposed to know everything, like God.

It is not possible to dispense with imagining an actor, or an author, for each discourse. Each discourse seems to start from a semblance/semblant. So we must make a semblance of having this author of discourse. However, this is merely the semblance of an identity. The master would be the author of the master discourse,

1 "Holding as true" refers to the Kantian expression *Für Wahr halten*, which entails for Kant essentially three types of approach to truth: knowledge, faith and opinion. In his book *Tenir pour Vrai*, Fierens proposes the addition of a fourth type of holding as true, namely, repression. (2020). Paris: Hermann. [Ed.'s comment].

DOI: 10.4324/9781003712480-33

the hysteric would be the author of the hysteric discourse, and so on. It seems that 'I am what I am.'

Perhaps it is important to take the semblance of each discourse into account. This is the Ego of each discourse. There would be a specific narcissism for each discourse: narcissism of the master, narcissism of the hysteric, narcissism of the academic, and narcissism of the analyst. Each of these does not just exist as a given reality, but entails the process leading to this semblance.

Ego or narcissism of the analyst	Ego or narcissism of the master
Ego or narcissism of the hysteric	Ego or narcissism of the academic

Too easily, we think that the Ego is determined by the mirror stage. The child would see its image in the mirror, every part of its body included in this image, and that is it. The Ego would be a great bag encompassing all the limbs and organs, body and mind.

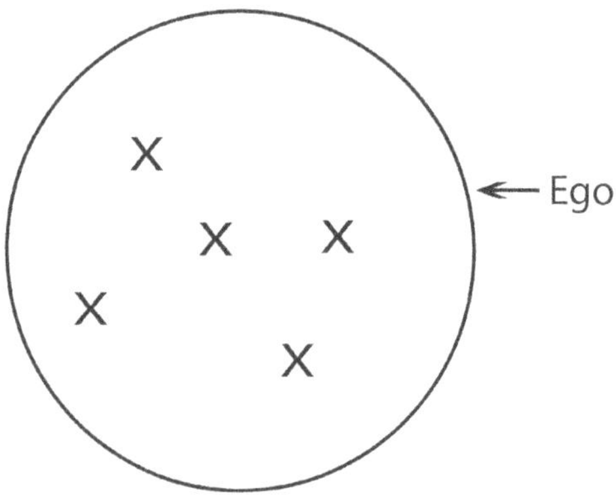

But the image in the mirror is not the Ego at all. It is impossible to think of, and to have, the Ego without the process in which it appears. Nevertheless, for each discourse one might think that the idea of its semblance is given as a Platonic idea, which would exist for all eternity. We would know what a master is, and what a hysteric, an academic, and an analyst are. We would have these four images, each of them encompassing the necessary traits to explain what a master is, what a hysteric is, and so on. Then everybody could take up these necessary traits to identify himself: to become a master, a hysteric, an academic, or an analyst. For each discourse, there would be a mirror stage founding the semblance of the discourse. So the discourse would be established by the narcissism of its semblance.

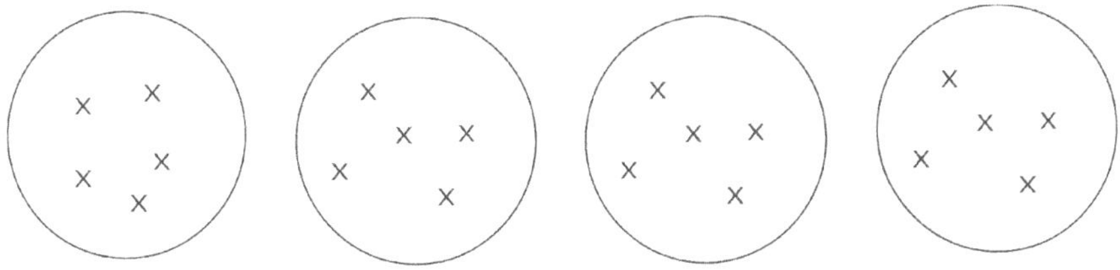

Ego of the analyst | Ego of the master | Ego of the hysteric | Ego of the academic

But first of all, the Ego and narcissism are a completely general process. Conversely, until now, they have been considered to be a big bag encompassing the compounds or the elements of the soul and of its specific forms—the master, the hysteric, the academic and the analyst.

In his introduction of the concept of narcissism, Freud emphasised the generality of this concept which is used for psychosis, neurosis, perversion, normality, and so on. 'I am what I am' and 'I love myself' are general, the general egotism or selfishness of human beings. To take into account the fact that love is always sexual, Freud termed it narcissism. So the term 'narcissism' came to describe the behaviour of an individual who treats his own body as his sexual object. Thus, narcissism is sexuality.

But what then is the difference between narcissism and more general autoeroticism of the libido? In the history of psychoanalysis, the specificity of narcissism in relation to autoeroticism is, from the outset, situated in the succession of stages. In the beginning, the Ego did not yet exist while the autoerotic drives were already in place. ". . . there must be something added to auto-erotism [. . .] in order to bring about narcissism."[2] This something is the place of the mirror stage. The mirror stage adds something—a bag perhaps—to autoeroticism, with the result that we now have the whole subject. Afterwards, starting from this whole narcissistic subject, it is possible to fall in love with something as another whole: with an object.

1. Autoeroticism	2. Narcissism Mirror stage	3. Love for an object

We are accustomed to understanding this addition as the purchase of the Ego as a bag that can contain the autoerotic drives and every part of the body and mind. We are accustomed to understanding the Ego as the container of the 'soul' in the second Freudian topography, or the structural model.[3] The Ego is then seen as the skin. This is the conception of the Skin-Ego following Didier Anzieu.

2 Freud, S. (1914c). *On Narcissism: An Introduction. SE XIV*. London: Hogarth Press, p. 77. Cited in Fierens, C. (2019). *The Soul of Narcissism*. M. G. Plastow (Trans.). London & New York: Routledge & Taylor & Francis Group, p. 32.

3 Here we use "soul", the literal translation of Freud's term *Seele*. In the English version of the *Standard Edition*, Strachey translates this as "psychic apparatus" [Trans.].

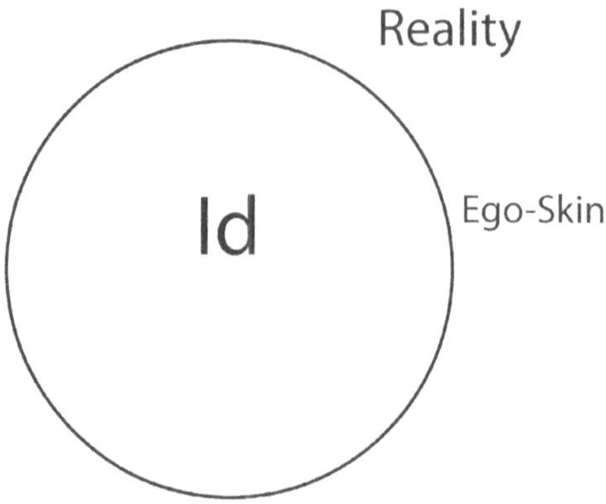

But the Ego is not such a bag. In his schemas, Freud did not situate the Ego as the skin of the soul, but in its centre.[4]

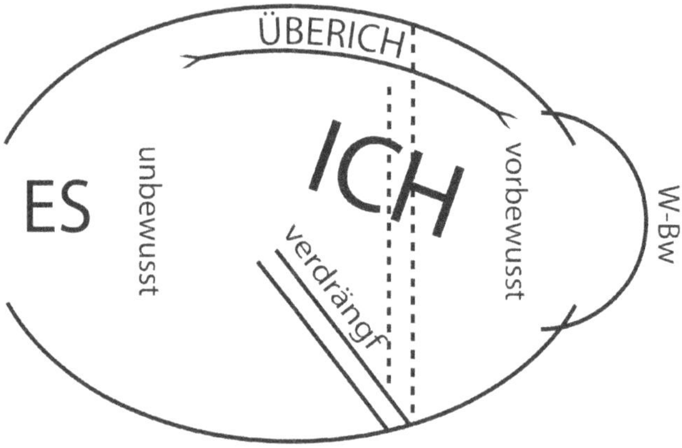

The Ego has to be developed (*entwickelt werden*) and its development is much more complex than the acquisition of a bag or of a skin, which would unite the different elements of body and mind.

The introduction of the concept 'narcissism' is not at all the introduction of a given synthesis of the psychic apparatus. Of course, if we had this synthesis, it would be easy to place each patient within the framework of this synthesis and its theory. But this is not the Freudian pathway. On the contrary, it begins with a

4 Freud, S. (1969). Neue Folge der Vorlesungen zur Einführung in die Psychoanalyse. GW XV: 85.

questioning, a questioning that goes on and on. The conception of narcissism is thus divided into two contradictory pathways. The first considers narcissism in accordance with a whole, with a synthesis in which you can situate and understand everything, and find the answer. The second sees narcissism in the development of a question. Both of these points of view seem to be merely theoretical. But each implies quite a different kind of practice.

Narcissism as a whole synthesis	Development or narcissism A questioning

Let us now start with the second point of view, the questioning one. Freud used the term 'narcissism' for the first time in his writing about Leonardo da Vinci.[5] The enigma of sexuality and the birth of a human being was very cumbersome for little Leonardo, all the more so since he was born out of wedlock to the notary of Vinci and a young peasant girl. He lived alone with his mother and, moreover, the legitimate wife of the notary remained childless. This situation appears to have exacerbated his questioning about the functioning of sexuality.

We can say that narcissism always occurs in the wake of the questioning of sexuality. Distinct from narcissism, autoerotism seems to go without question. It works as it works without any reflexion, without any thinking, without any feedback.

The questioning of sexuality begins with the statement that it does not work. Thus, there is an enigma. Yet, to think about this failure, this lack, this enigma implies that it was possible that, 'once upon a time,' everything was in order, without any lack, without any questioning. So, starting from lack, from the enigma of sexuality and castration, the reflexion of the little child looks for a construction in which everything was okay. He can imagine himself as the perfect child. Once upon a time, he was His Majesty the Baby, endlessly loved by his parents: that is the Ideal Ego. This imagining is put in the past. He was, and that is the guarantee that he can find this perfection once again.

Now, with this imagining of a wonderland, it becomes possible to look for an answer in the future. Starting from this past perfection, the Ideal Ego (that is, an Ego), he looks forward to retrieving it in the future, not just as an imaginary one, but as a symbolic accomplishment of his life. That is the Ego Ideal (that is, an Ideal).

5 Freud, S. (1910). Leonardo da Vinci and a memory of his childhood. SE XI: 57.

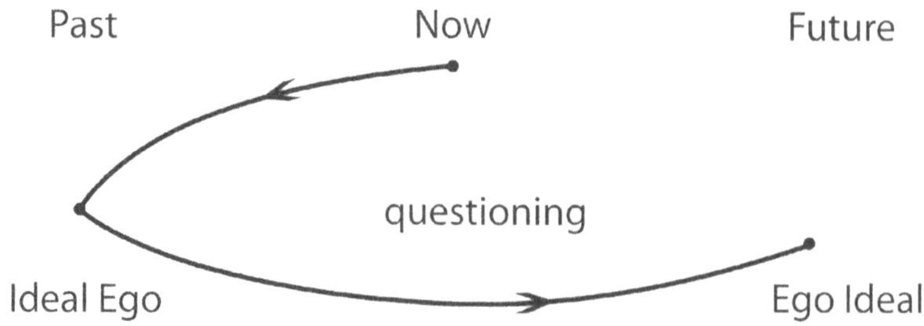

In this schema, the Ego exists only in the movement that entails the Ideal Ego in the past as well as the Ego Ideal in the future. We must consider the Ego in the whole process of its development. Here I quote from Freud's essay, "On Narcissism": "The development of the Ego consists in a departure from primary narcissism [i.e. the Ideal Ego] and gives rise to a vigorous attempt to recover that state [i.e. in the Ego Ideal]."[6]

To form this Ideal Ego, this primary narcissism—which is not real but imaginary—the process implicates the control and the mastering of each element at stake in the structure, in other words, the synthesis of everything. So the Ideal Ego is presented as a whole. This is the image of the Ego in the mirror stage. It is the spherical mirror in Lacan's optical schema: each flower seems to be in the vase, and each part of the body and mind seems to be in the Ideal Ego, but this is only a semblance.

This image, this Ideal Ego, does not exist except in the process. If we consider this image as the essence of the Ego or of narcissism (first conception of narcissism), we miss the point of the Ego and narcissism as the process which also includes the symbolic movement towards the future of the Ego Ideal (second conception of narcissism). Thus, Lacan has to place a second mirror in his optical schema in order to engage the movement. The first mirror has no momentum at all.

If we think within the first conception (without the process), we will always hold it as true, and we will be satisfied, because narcissism implies this stage. It will seem enough to classify our narcissistic patient in the imaginary field. But here we miss the process of narcissism itself, which is never simple and which always implies an indefinite search for the Ego Ideal. We can hear this process in every form of narcissism. It is not always conspicuous, and we have to look for it. But it exists, and this is the only way to enter into the movement of psychoanalysis.

Such development of the Ego is always running from the beginning of life to its end. The development of the Ego is never finished, except in death. The topography of narcissism is therefore stretched between the Ideal Ego and the Ego Ideal. This explains the birth of Freud's structural model, which comes after the first model—or the topographical model—and also after the model of narcissism.

So, let us come to the second model, namely the structural model with the Id [Es], the Ego [*Ich*] and the Superego [*Überich*]. Here, the development of the Ego is in

6 Freud, S. (1914*c*). On narcissism: An introduction. SE XIV: 100 [my emphasis].

the centre. But the Id takes part in this process: the development of the Ego begins long before the consciousness of the Ego. The movement starting from the questioning—going back to imagining a perfect whole in the past and trying to retrieve it in the future—is always at stake. The Id must be considered part of this structure. It is not a bag of given elements, but is the structure of the Ego's movement prior to the Ego, prior to the consciousness of the Ego. And the Superego [*Überich*] is not only an instance that is imposed upon the Ego, but that which allows the functioning of the Ego, quite similar to the Ego Ideal. In considering the development of the Ego, we do not have a given Ego, but the formation of an always divided Ego, and twice divided. It is divided between the conscious process (Ego) and the unconscious one (Id), and divided between the Ideal Ego (Ego) and the Ego Ideal (Superego).

We cannot analyse the Id, except if we let it work. And then it becomes the Ego: *Wo Es war, soll Ich werden*: "where the Id was, there Ego shall be."[7] This is quite practical and implies the ethical dimension of the unconscious passing through the Ego.

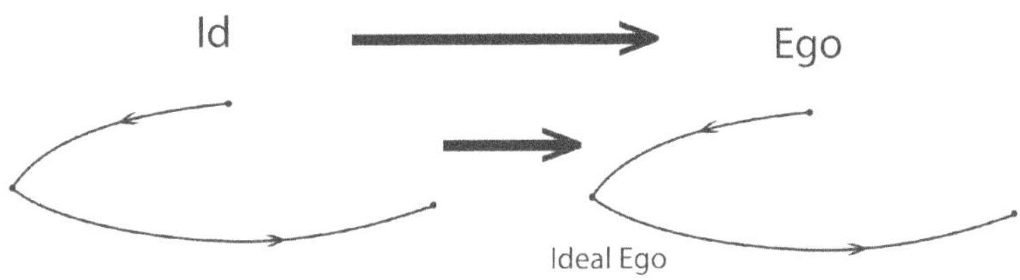

We shall return later to the division between the Id and the Ego. Let us now consider the second division between a lower stage (let us say the Ego and its fantasy, the Ideal Ego) and an upper stage (let us say the Ego Ideal or the Superego). 'Stage' is the translation of the German *Stufe*, which always entails the special opposition of high and low and not so much the temporal opposition between before and after. The high position of the upper stage also implies the ethical dimension (what is to be done), but it seems quite outside the ego, which only seems factual (what actually or really is).

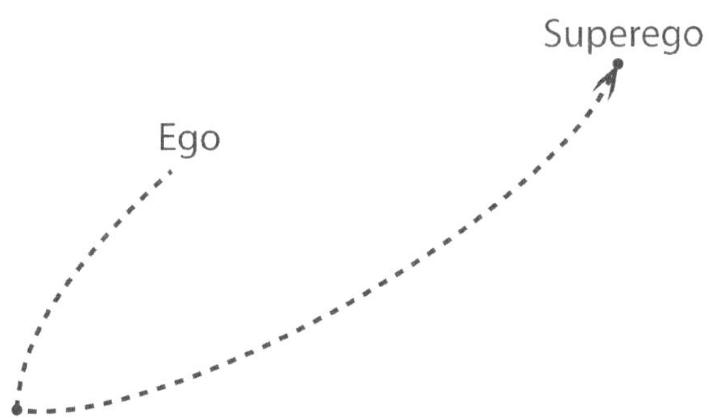

7 Freud, S. (1933). New introductory lectures on psycho-analysis. SE XXII: 80.

With this division between Ego and Superego or Ego Ideal, Freud can explain the very existence of two main kinds of groups: church and army. In his work, *Group Psychology and the Analysis of the Ego*, the psychology of the group in general is explained through the analysis of the Ego in its two components: the lower one (the Ego) and the upper one (the Superego).[8] So we can understand each group—army, church and psychoanalytic group—as the result of the process of narcissism or of the Ego's development.

The actual Ego seeks an object in the external world that could tally sufficiently with its Ideal Ego, that is, with what was supposed to have been perfect in the past. He then puts this in the place of its aim, of its Ego Ideal, and identifies himself with this object. The object could be a person or an abstract idea. In any case, it takes the place of the genuine Ego Ideal in this process of identification.

When we have a large number of people who are identified with, for example, Christ, as their Ego Ideal, we have the church. When they are identified with the nation to be defended or extended, as their Ego Ideal, we have an army. When they are identified with the so-called psychoanalytic cause, with a famous psychoanalyst or with a collection of big idealistic ideas, we have the psychoanalytic group. The structure in any case is the same. The different Egos delegate all of their power to the embodiment of their Ideal Ego in a common leader. Whether this is a person or an ideal does not matter. For every type of group, everybody is identified with this leader, with the Führer.

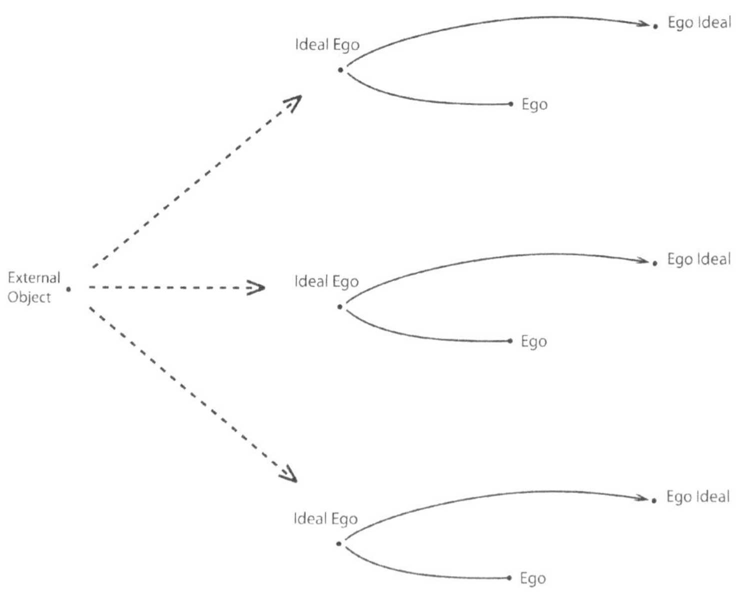

8 Freud, S. (1921c). Group psychology and the analysis of the ego. SE XVIII: 65.

At the end of Chapter VIII in *Group Psychology and the Analysis of the Ego*, Freud provides approximately the same schema of the group in his work, but in the reverse order. Here I place it in its correct order to let it be understood that, each time, the Ego calls upon an object that is already there, in order to place it as the aim of its life which is ahead, in the future, as his Ego Ideal, giving substance and consistency to his soul.

Identification

Identification is always identification with something that can take the place of an Ego Ideal. With identification it is possible to find other people who have undertaken to find a similar object representing their Ego Ideal and, so, loving the same object, to form a group. A group consists of a number of people with the same representative of their Ego Ideal. Identification, in its structure, leads directly to the formation of a group, whether big or small.

But what is the mechanism of identification? We must eat the elephant one bite at a time. It is the same for identification. We must first identify ourselves with a trait, a unary trait. Then we can add a second trait, and so on, until it seems that we have reached an identification with the whole person. But it is always taken bit by bit, piece by piece, bite by bite, as for the elephant. So for Freud, the process of identification always seems to start with oral consumption.

Nowadays, the psychoanalytic field seems to be focused on two points: the identification of the analysand at the end of analysis, and the formation of psychoanalytic groups. Both points are focused on narcissism as a result, as a synthesis, and not on narcissism as a process, as the development of the Ego.

However, firstly, we must say that the end of analysis is not the identification of the analysand. But to eliminate identification he ought not look for the implementation of the Ego Ideal. He need not become stuck on an identity. He has to move on, to always become other. Secondly, we must say, following Lacan, that there is no psychoanalytic group at all. The members of a cartel meet with each other, not in so far as they have the same Ego Ideal, but because they can occupy different positions in relation to each other.

For the connection between sexuality and narcissism, we cannot remain stuck in the first conception of narcissism (as a whole, a bag). Yes, this is the first pathway to understanding sexuality. Yes, as they say, narcissism is the great reservoir of libido, the libido tank, or perhaps, the water tank. But this is a buffer tank, and we must understand the very process of this buffer.

Let us now start again from the development of the Ego. Initially, we will consider the Ego Ideal. For the reflexion of the Ego, we have to build a possibility, the possibility of mastering everything—that is, the Ideal Ego—but this is necessarily included in the implementation of an Ego Ideal. The possibility of the Ideal Ego does not exist outside the prospect of the movement of the Ego, its necessity to look forward to recovering the imaginary perfection. This seems to imply the embodiment of the Ego Ideal, namely, the aforementioned leader.

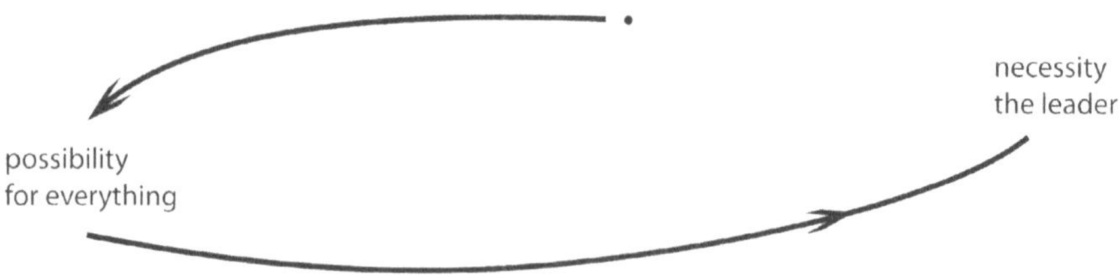

First of all, it seems that the movement, which is always based on sexuality, can be summarised in the imaginary world of the Ideal Ego. Everything can tally with this perfection. "Everything is Phi of x:" first masculine formula of sexuation. But secondly, it implies the necessity, the need, for implementing it, namely in the exception or in the leader, who provides the real boundaries of this imaginary world: "there exists an x not Phi of x," second masculine formula of sexuation.

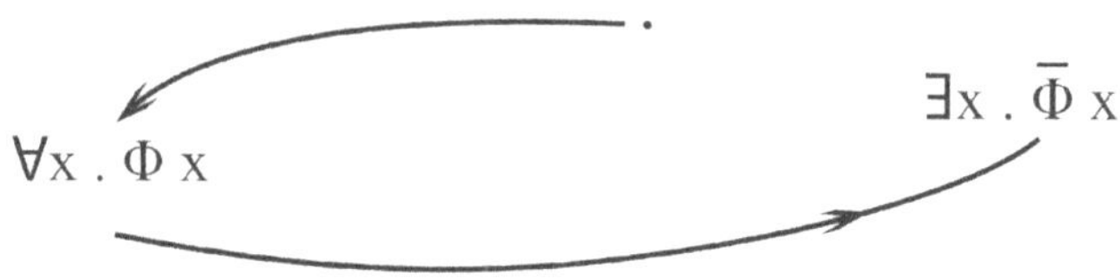

So, the development of the Ego—of narcissism—seems to tally perfectly with the masculine formulae of sexuation. Masculine sexuation would therefore be the essence of narcissism. And sexuation in general would be the masculine form, the phallic one.

In this schema, we have forgotten the starting point, that is, the questioning. It is always the same mistake which leads us to the first conception of narcissism, or to focusing on the group, or to the conception of analysis as identification, or to sexuality as a masculine one. We act as if we really had the Ideal Ego or the good functioning of the phallic function. We act as if we really had the Ego Ideal in the person of a saint, a leader or a founder. But we do not have the reality of the Ideal Ego, or the reality of the Ego Ideal. We have simply constructed the possibility of an Ideal Ego and the good functioning of the so-called phallus that always, sooner or later, recedes, retreats and shrinks. We have simply built the necessity of a hero as a template for our narcissism and our Ego Ideal. We are holding these points as true. But they are not the truth.

Thus, the development of narcissism does not consist in the results of the possibility of the phallic function, or in the necessity of the exception, but in returning to the very question at the beginning of the process. There is absolutely no leader, no saint, no implementation of the Ego Ideal ("there does not exist an x not Phi of x:" first feminine formula of sexuation). Moreover, the possibility or the presupposition of a perfect phallic functioning is simply a fiction that sometimes works but not always. Not all can be put in the phallic function (second feminine formula of sexuation).

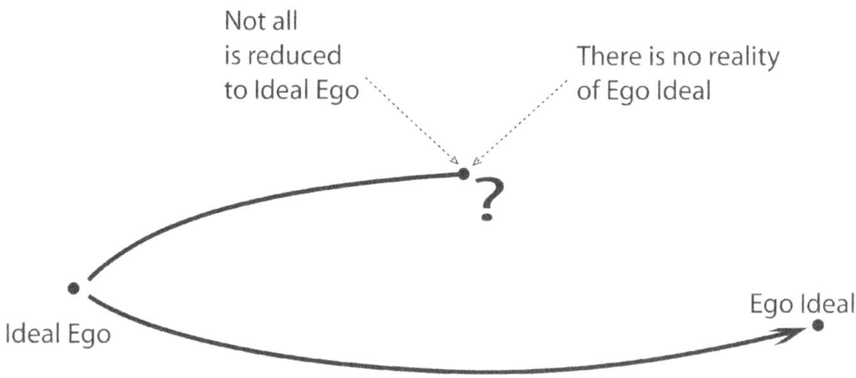

If we take into account not only the results of narcissism but also its very process, it becomes conspicuous that this entails not only the Ideal Ego as a whole or a bag. The aim is also to implement the Ego Ideal, and much more. There is no real implementation of this Ego Ideal, which always remains an ideal. It is impossible to include everything in the Ideal Ego. These remarks again lead us to a questioning. The development of the Ego never ends. We have to start the whole process again and again in a roundabout with the Ideal Ego, the Ego Ideal, with the inexistence of the Ego Ideal and with what escapes from the Ideal Ego. The development of the process entails the roundabout of the four formulae of sexuation.

What is sexuation? Is this the same as sexuality? Sexuality is supposed to be given, a given reality. But we know that such a given sexuality does not exist. It always depends on its own experience, which is always a questioning one, the questioning which is the starting point of narcissism. With this questioning, it implies doing something (doing something with words). As in the Cartesian Ego, this does not appear without the questioning of hyperbolic doubt. Then it becomes crucial to understand that we have to do sexuality, and not just to do something with a supposed given sexuality. That is sexuation: manufacturing or producing sex, following the very development of the Ego, following the soul of narcissism.

I said following. But is it not the contrary? Narcissism follows sexuation, as we could see in the sequence of autoeroticism narcissism. Here it is important to see that the structure of sexuation (autoeroticism) and of narcissism is quite the same. The structure of sexuation is precisely what is at stake in the Freudian Id. But we cannot bring about direct access to sexuation, to autoeroticism or to the Id, without the help of narcissistic questioning. So, from an ontological and theoretical point of view, we must consider that the structure of the Id and sexuation exists prior to the development of the Ego. But from a practical point of view, we must deal directly with narcissism, and that is the case in the practice of analysis.

The practice of psychoanalysis in light of sexuation and narcissism

In a footnote of 1924, Freud writes that the acknowledgment of the Oedipus complex is the shibboleth that distinguishes supporters and enemies of psychoanalysis. What does this mean? Freud's analysis of the Wolf Man emphasises that it is not sufficient to say that the method of psychoanalysis is the method of free associations. With free speech alone, it might be considered sufficient to tell the analyst anything. But the analyst must sustain evenly-poised attention to the map of that which occurs in the mind of the analysand: unconscious, preconscious and conscious. And this second rule of psychoanalytic practice introduces something quite new: that childhood sexuality is always and primarily what is at stake. This is not simply as a consequence of the present imagination of the analysand or of the analyst—as proposed by Jung and Adler—but as the very beginning of his psychic life, which always remains involved in the present, in the transference. We say "childhood sexuality": "sexuality," because sexuality continually remains at stake in any interest which enlivens life, and "child," because the beginning is never lost, and we have to continually begin again. In order to effect an analysis of an adult neurotic, we must take into account his or her development, which began much earlier. We must take into account his endless childhood neurosis. We must go back to his Oedipus complex, that is, to the beginning of sexual structuration.

However, this so-called analysis is not just an observation. The analysand and the analyst are both involved in the transference. It would be an oversimplification to reduce this transference to the division of roles: the analysand would be the child and the analyst would be the father or the mother. Essentially, it is not a matter of roles or functions, but a matter of questioning. It is important to shift away from these roles to arrive at a questioning which is fundamental. Here, "fundamental" has a dual meaning. Firstly, it refers to a questioning about the fundaments of human life. What is life? What is death? What is sexuality? What am I? Secondly, it is a founding questioning, as such the process which establishes and supports the development of the Ego and its life. This we have seen starting from the central point, going back to the imaginary Ideal Ego and then looking forward to the so-called recovery of a satisfaction.

If we failed to recognise such questioning, we would be, following Freud, the enemies of psychoanalysis. We must recognise the importance of narcissism as not simply the dead end of a forgotten process, but as the possible implementation of the fundamental questioning of human beings. Such questioning is the process of sexuation, which goes much further than a given sexuality. To practise psychoanalysis, we must not only practise the two masculine formulae of sexuation—which seem to tally with the usual concept of narcissism—but also the four formulae with the feminine formulae endlessly relaunching the infinite process of narcissism.

How can one work with the formulae of sexuation? Starting from narcissism as a result—not as a process—we are accustomed to acting in the framework of the structural model, the division between the Ego and the Superego (or Ego Ideal). We then look forward to finding supports, assistance, as well as for the identification of the Ego, as for the formation of a group around the Ego Ideal. Analysis is running after the identification of the patient's Ego and is standardised with the psychoanalytic group around a psychoanalytic ideal. From that point of view, any discourse starts from its agent—its semblance—and organises a social bond, a particular group.

But development of Ego, sexuality and sexuation do not exist outside the movement of questioning which is the core, the soul of narcissism (as is obvious with Leonardo da Vinci). Firstly, we do not have the Ego. We do not have a master, a hysteric, an academic, or a psychoanalyst, but questioning without any support. We must think through any discourse with this questioning about truth outside of any support. We must think through the discourses following the questioning of the truth, through the different kinds of holding as true. Such questioning, which is revealed in the development of the Ego, exists prior to any support. We must come back to the first division of the Ego, the division between the Ego and the Id. This is the core of the unconscious, which is always working, always dynamic.

The practice of psychoanalysis awakens and sparks the movement of the unconscious, which is the roundabout of the formulae of sexuation, revealed in the process of narcissism. But this process must be brought back to its roots—to childhood sexuality—which is already a full sexuation. "What is a child?" asks Michael Plastow.

Thus, transference is no longer a matter of people or of the Ego, but a matter of sexuation inside the dynamic of the unconscious Id. Through any form of narcissism, it is possible to read this dynamic and to let it work, and then to allow a new form of the Ego to appear. This is not equal to a given being, but it is working, always in development. It is here that we find the field of creation.

Chapter 27

Symptom and sinthome

Christian Fierens

"Symptom" is the generally accepted spelling of a word that in Greek, etymologically speaking, means coincidence. Here, unconscious desire and preconscious defence merge to form the symptom. This is the 'common' spelling but an academic one, dating from the Renaissance (re-birth). If Lacan had wished to go back to the older spelling—"sinthome"—prior to its Hellenisation, it was not precisely from an academic point of view, but rather, to catch the thing at its first emergence, in its first origin, in its first birth. The first spelling, "sinthome," entails "sin," that is, a first and fundamental lack, a first failure before everything else. And this will completely change the practice of psychoanalysis.

We know that the practice of psychoanalysis awakens and sparks the movement of the unconscious and the roundabout of the formulae of sexuation, both of which are at stake in the process of narcissism. This process must be brought back to its roots, to its first beginnings, to childhood sexuality, which is already a full sexuation with the four formulae.

The process of narcissism does not begin with the Ego, but in the Id, with a questioning which attempts to enclose everything (that will become the Ideal Ego: "for all x phi of x"), through given limits (that will be represented by an Ego Ideal: "there exists an x not phi of x"). But such an Ego Ideal does not exist. There are holes in the fence: "there does not exist an x not phi of x." There does not exist such a true Ego Ideal. Moreover, it is not true that we could enclose everything in the enclosure: "notall phi of x." With the two feminine formulae of sexuation, supposing a failure, a "sin," the process of narcissism is indefinitely relaunched. There is another attempt to enclose everything including this "notall," and so on.

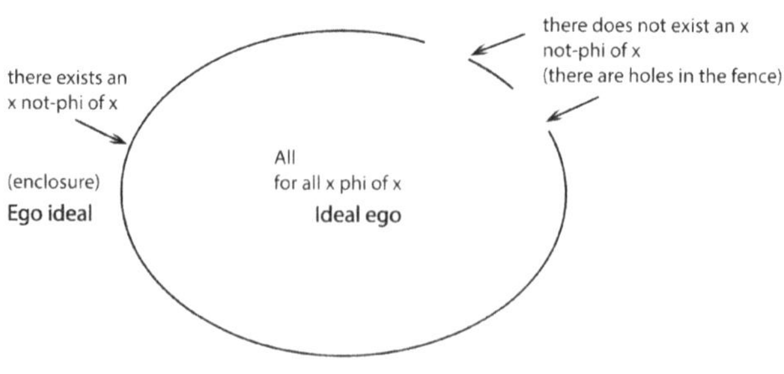

DOI: 10.4324/9781003712480-34

How can we locate this roundabout of the four formulae of sexuation in the very practice of psychoanalysis, in the treatment of the symptom? First, we will consider treatment of the symptom according to the Freudian conception. Secondly, I will outline the conception of the sinthome following the fundamental sin, following the sin according to the Lacanian conception. And, finally, we will extract the relevant consequences for a new psychoanalytic practice.

The Freudian conception of the symptom is comprised of three points. First, the symptom is a compromise. It is composed. Thus, it would be possible to analyse it and to find its components. The treatment is an analysis. Secondly, the symptom takes place in a process of relaunching. The treatment is then a relaunching. Thirdly, the symptom in itself is a construction. The treatment is then the construction of a new psychic reality.

Let us explore these points in more detail. Firstly, the symptom is a compromise between an unconscious sexual drive and a preconscious defence against this drive. These two forces are equal, but are pushing in opposite directions. Each force is holding the other. Nothing is moving. The hysterical crisis does not change anything, the obsessive symptom is inhibition, and the phobic symptom is stuck in its treatment of anguish. Contrary to other formations of the unconscious that are easily forgotten, such symptoms insist and persist for years and years. With the method of free association it would be possible to analyse, to disentangle, this compromise, and to separate the meaning of the unconscious drive and the meaning of the preconscious defence against it. Following this analysis, it would be easy for the analysand—outside or after the genuine analysis—to make the best choices for his life. In chapter XVII of his lectures on psychoanalysis,[1] Freud dealt with the meaning of the symptom.

Secondly, the relaunching. After two beautiful examples of this type of analysis, Freud arrives directly at a worrying assessment. He generally fails to explain what he calls "typical symptoms." With his own method of free association, which involves looking for meaning, he does not succeed in telling us why the patient specifically produces a hysterical symptom, an obsessive symptom, or a phobic one. This is very disturbing because it appears to be a complete setback for interpretation. In *The Interpretation of Dreams*, Freud had already encountered a similar problem. With so-called "typical dreams"—dreams of nakedness, dreams of death of beloved people, dreams where the dreamer is hovering or floating in the air, dreams of exams—Freud fails to find an interpretation through his own method. He proposes a pragmatic solution—symbolic interpretation. Mind! This seems to contradict his own method. Nevertheless, Freud uses just one symbol, and this is the phallic one. More precisely, it is always the phallic function that is at stake. This function is not a usual function going from a given point to a given point.

1 Freud, S. (1916–1917). Lecture XVII: The sense of symptoms. In: *Introductory Lectures on Psycho-Analysis (Part III)*. SE XVI: 257–272.

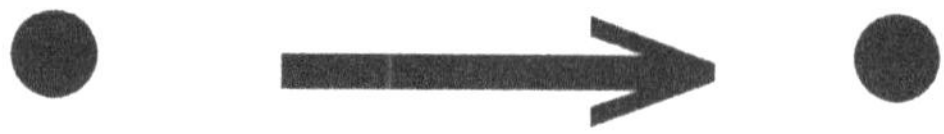

With the phallic function, it starts from what we do not know. It starts outside any fixed point. We are taken in a movement without any given reference point, and we do not reach a final point. This is a relaunching function. We can write it thus: arrow dot arrow.

The typical dream is always considered in this process of relaunching, beyond any meaning of the dream. And each dream, with its possible meaning, must be placed in this revival. It is the same for the typical symptom. Its issues are always to be placed within the process of relaunching beyond any meaning. So, the hysterical symptom tries to relaunch desire through the questioning of any stable point, and this keeps desire outside of satisfaction. Desire is unsatisfied. Thus, the phobic symptom tries to foresee, to provide, and to prevent the anguish of desire, and the relaunching is then scheduled in a closed space. Desire is prevented. Thus, the obsessive symptom perpetually tries to explain the relaunching point. Remaining in this central point, it loses the possibility of desire itself. Desire is impossible.

If the symptom is to be taken up in a process of relaunching, it must be understood not as a given reality, but rather, within the very process of its formation, of its development. Freud himself cannot be satisfied with his chapter XVII on the meaning of symptoms.[2] He must delve further and arrive at the topic of chapter XXIII of the same lectures on psychoanalysis, "The paths to the formation of symptoms," or in a better translation, "The ways of symptom formation."[3]

We arrive here at the third Freudian point: construction of psychical reality. Chapter XXIII of the lectures on psychoanalysis responds to the end of chapter XVII, which outlines the failure to explain symptoms in terms of meaning. Firstly, it seems here that everything in the symptom starts with sexuality and with a failure in the sexual field. There is always a more or less important failure: there is a trauma. For everybody, the encounter with sexuality is always traumatic. In the beginning, it would have been the reality or the real of sexuality.

Secondly, upon this reality, psychic life would always build fantasies, phantasms. Upon the primary real, the imaginary would build a new world, let us say a world of symptoms entailing not just the real, but also the imaginary. On the first

2 Freud, S. (1916–1917). Lecture XVII.

3 Freud, S. (1916–1917). Lecture XXIII: The paths to the formation of symptoms. In: *Introductory Lectures on Psycho-Analysis (Part III)*. SE XVI: 358–377.

level, on the first floor, we would have the real world or reality. On the second level, we would have the imaginary of the psychic world. We think that these two worlds are separated: what reality is, cannot not be psychic imagination, and what psychic imagination is, cannot be reality. Nevertheless, the symptom seems to be a mixture of reality and psychic: a 'psychical reality.' This is quite difficult to conceive of because 'reality' and 'psychical' are conflicting and contradictory.

Then, the so-called psychotherapist arrives and begins to comment on the situation. That is the third level, the top floor, a symbolic one. But he speaks upon the real and upon the imaginary of the symptom. And it is impossible to change anything of the symptom simply by speaking about and upon it. The symptom would resist any kind of psychotherapy. The so-called psychotherapist cannot be a therapist at all. The talking cure would be only a smooth talking, without any effect either on reality or on the imaginary.

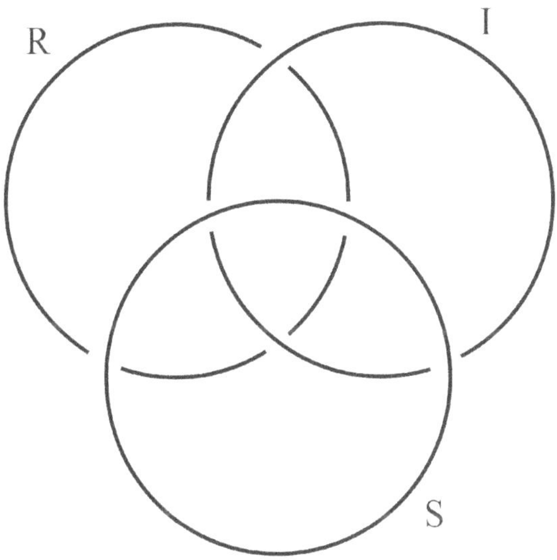

With these three separate levels—real, imaginary and symbolic—it is impossible to think of the efficiency of psychoanalysis. It is also impossible to think about formation of the symptom. And yet, we have symptoms and we have the effectiveness of psychoanalysis. As a matter of fact, symptoms, and with them, psychoanalysis, invent a formation through which a particular production of the symbolic—this is not just a comment—would be the basis of the real and the imaginary, of reality and the psychic. This basis is so-called 'psychical reality.'[4]

4 Lacan, J. (1974–1975). *Le séminaire livre XXII*, R.S.I. Unpublished manuscript, session of 14/01/75. See Fierens, C. (2018). *Lecture du sinthome*. Toulouse: ERES, pp. 20–36.

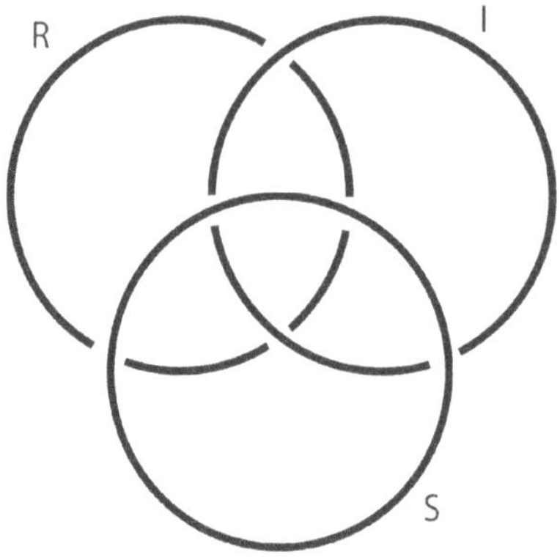

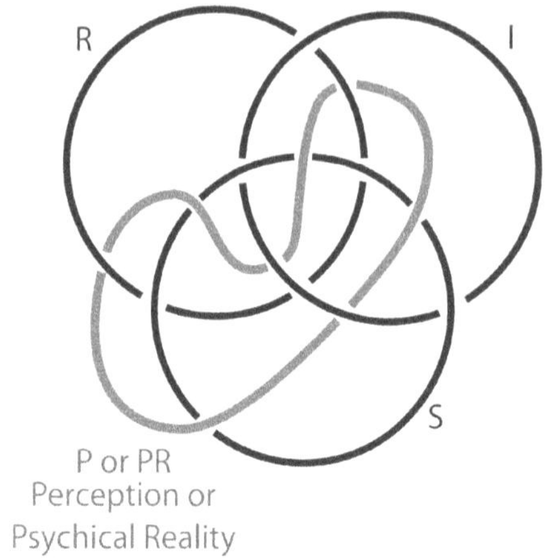

Psychical reality is constructed upon the symbolic. It depends on it. And upon itself—upon psychical reality. The real and the imaginary are constructed. They do not exist except by depending on the 'psychical reality.' The symptom is not a reality, nor is it a psychic imagination. Rather, it is a 'psychical reality,' which sustains each part of the reality and the imagination of the patient.

It is very important to understand such a structure of the symptom, because this provides access to the very functioning of transference in the psychoanalytic treatment. Transference and symptoms do exactly the same thing: they construct a psychical reality upon the symbolic process and, with it, at the same time, they sustain interest in reality and the invention of the imagination. Transference and the symptom have exactly the same structure. In this sense, the psychoanalyst takes part in the symptom. We have seen the importance of the symptom and transference in the framework of the trilogy—real, imaginary and symbolic—and there is also a fourth element that is always in formation, in development.

We can assume now that the development of psychical reality occurs after a failure: after a failure of the symbolic to change anything in the real and in the imaginary, or after a failure of the real which had no grounds at all. This double failure entails, then, a double questioning which is already at stake in the questioning of narcissism. How is it possible to change the world with a mere ideal, the Ego Ideal, which does not switch to reality? How is it possible to take the real into account, when already, everything starts with the imagination of the Ego, of the Ideal Ego, with so-called narcissism?

The answer to this double questioning is in the movement of the questions which constitute the development of the Ego. Firstly, it would be possible to change reality with the Ego Ideal, as long as we have its embodiment in a leader or a founder of a new world ("there exists an x not phi of x") and we have the identification with him in any group. Secondly, with him, it would be possible to give a foundation of reality ("all x phi of x"). But these answers of the two masculine formulae of sexuation are insufficient, because they go forward as if the Ego Ideal and its embodiment in the leader were a true reality, independent of the questioning. So, the pathway for this double questioning entails not only the two masculine formulae of sexuation, which give answers, but also the feminine ones, which keep the questioning alive: "there does not exist a leader up to the Ego Ideal" and "not all can be contained in the imagination of the Ideal Ego."

The questioning inherent in psychic reality is the questioning inherent in the development of the Ego. It is the structure of narcissism and of the Id. This must be understood through the roundabout of the four formulae of sexuation. The formation of psychical reality is sexuation. And Freud called this the fundamental phantasm, fundamental in a double sense. One, it is the grounds of psychic reality. And two, it raises fundamental questions: what is life? What is love? What is death? What are sexuation and castration? This is also at stake in the symptom, like it is in the transference. With transference, psychoanalysis is going in exactly the same way—the same method—as the symptom, hopefully a better way.

Where can we find this "better way?" Here we must start at the very beginning, that is, before the consciousness of the Ego: that would be the Id. And we must start before any academic explanation of it in the meaning of the symptom as a compromise, as is obvious in the Greek etymology of "symptom." We must start with the sinthome.

The Lacanian conception of the sinthome

We can find something of the structure of psychical reality in Freud, in chapter XXIII of his lectures in psychoanalysis.[5] Lacan offered the graph of this structure in his *R.S.I.* seminar as the nomination of the real. This means that we do not have the real: its grounds are lacking, but with the help of the symbolic, we can manage to give it a foundation. We can also think that we do not have the symbolic: its grounds are lacking, but we can manage to find its foundation. And the same for the imaginary, a foundation of the imaginary. We would start from a real conception of psychoanalysis (that is Freud), from a symbolic conception (that would be Lacan) or from an imaginary conception (that would be Melanie Klein, for example). Each time, we would encounter the lack of a precise form, the lack of the real, the lack of the symbolic, the lack of the imaginary. And afterwards we would have to repair it or find a substitute, a foundation or a so-called nomination.

But, according to Lacan, the sinthome does not start with one or other dimension, and afterwards we would take stock that it fails. We do not have these dimensions, as the manner of approaching psychoanalysis. The lack is a priori, before

5 Freud, S. (1916–1917). Lecture XXIII.

the appearance of everything. This is the "sin" of sinthome, the primary failure. However, in our busy world, we possess an innumerable quantity of things. More and more. Of course, it is possible to think about a lot of lacks, a lot of failures. But with these innumerable lacks, we do not reach the a priori lack, the primary failure or the original sin of the sinthome.

Before we answer the question—how can we take stock of this primary failure?—I emphasise the importance of this radical lack. Firstly, the meaning of the symptom is not sufficient to treat it and does not reach the essence of the symptom. Secondly, the relaunching of the symptom supposes being able to rid oneself of the static dots and to begin with the moving arrow, which entails a radical lack. Thirdly, the formation of the symptom implies a void, a lack prior to the formation. Now, how can we approach this lack?

This is the very questioning at stake: why is there anything rather than nothing? A thing or nothing? A thing or lack?

According to Lacan, his only invention is the invention of the object *a*, which leads to a questioning: is it nothing or anything? Such affirmation seems strange because Freud had already emphasised the oral object, the anal object, and the scopic object, and the voice was well known in philosophy and in literature. The Lacanian invention does not consist in repeating these forms—oral, anal, scopic and voice—but in the manner of understanding the articulations of these different modalities of the same object *a*, of the same question: anything or nothing? And that will lead us to the very lack, to the original sin, the primary failure as an introduction to the sinthome.

Firstly, the manner of thinking nothing. We can have the idea of something which is not to be found in reality. There is nothing. For instance, the little baby can have the idea of an almighty breast, giving all satisfaction. But there is nothing of this kind, and that is the oral object. We already encounter this structure today. We have the idea of an Ego Ideal, but there is nothing of a true embodiment of this ideal. Furthermore, we have the idea of a perfect real, a perfect symbolic, a perfect imaginary, but there are necessary failures in each.

There is nothing of this purity in them. Each time, it is the same structure as the oral object. The treatment would be to find a substitute.

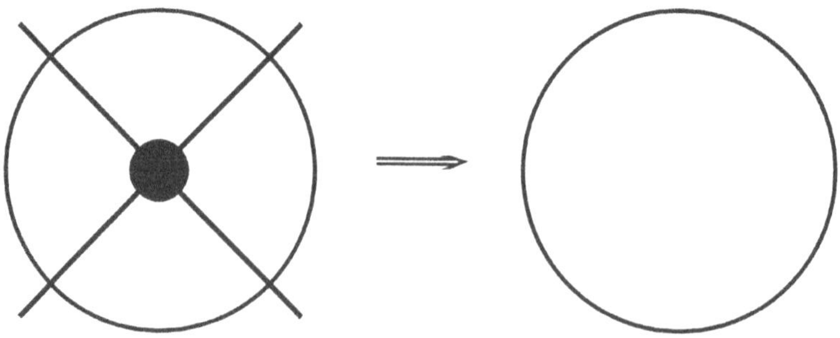

Second manner of thinking nothing. We can construct a "nothing" while opposing two forces equal in their degree but opposite in their direction. For instance, the baby can release a poo as a gift of love and at the same time as a weapon of hate. With regard to the balance between love and hate, the poo is zero. But in the anal stage it has its consequences. The parents are invited to deal with it. This is the very structure of the original repression. The quantity of the preconscious defence is identical to the quantity of the unconscious drive, but in the opposite direction. The result is an inhibition. Nothing moves in the external world, but inside it is quite moving. Moreover, poo is also called a "motion." This was the general meaning of the Freudian symptom as a compromise. It would be possible to disentangle these two forces. This is an analysis.

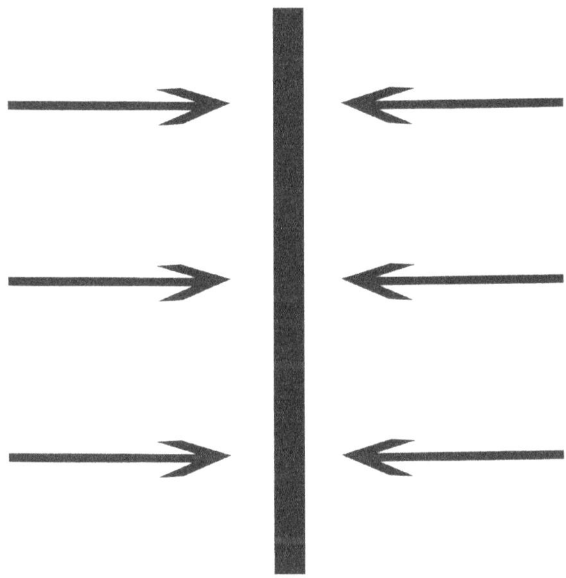

Third manner of thinking nothing. We can construct a map to encompass each object in our world. We can imagine a God's eye that can see everything. But this mapping necessarily entails a failure. Everything is lacking in this abstract map. In other words, in every vision of the world we encounter a blind spot. But this is not simply a limited spot. It is the gap between the abstraction of vision, of understanding, and the concrete object which escapes vision. This is the scopic object. We have already encountered this in the schema of psychical reality, as well as in similar schemas of different types of foundation or nomination. This type of mapping is a first type of topology—outside practice—and is not the true sense of psychoanalytic topology, even if it is the common presentation of topology in the psychoanalytic field today.

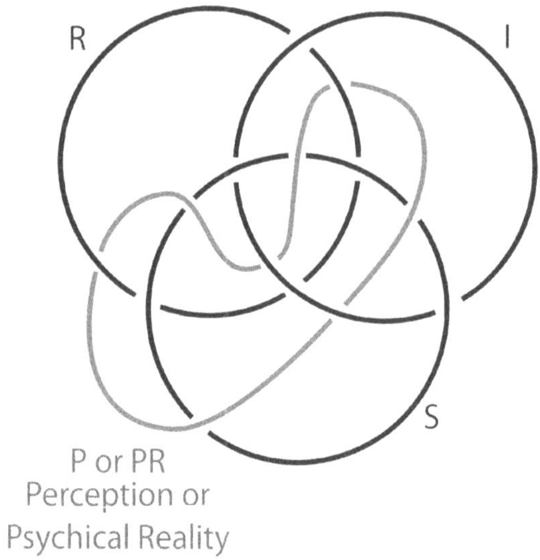

Fourth manner of thinking nothing. I have no schema at all to represent the fourth kind of object *a*, because this is precisely what contradicts the very conditions of any representation, the very conditions of any sensible experience. It is a radical nothing. As it cannot be seen, it is not the scopic object. But it cannot be heard either. It is the voice as silence.

We have already encountered a hint towards this radical nothing. In his practice, Freud encountered silence when he had to deal with typical symptoms, as well as with typical dreams. The very conditions of the psychoanalytic process—free associations—radically fail, and there is silence. Of course, the analyst might insist on beginning again with associations. Or better, as Freud suggests, he could say: "You are thinking about me, the analyst." But what does this mean? If the analysand is actually thinking about the person of the analyst, the issue is not so much the particularity of the analyst. It makes no sense to attempt to retrieve the pathway of associations and meanings about these particularities, which could evoke the father, the mother, or other people in the analysand's story. No! The importance of the analyst in this lack of associations is not at all the person of the analyst. The issue at stake here is the very function of the analyst as such. And this function is precisely to keep the place, the semblance place of the *object a* in its fully developed structure, its fourth form, the invocative object, or the radical nothing outside of any meaning.

But here psychoanalytic practice seems to be completely nihilistic. Or humbug, if you try to disavow it for your own interests. Whilst dealing with this radical nothing, however, Freud was neither nihilistic nor humbug. He introduced the relaunching of the phallic function. And with the introduction of the fourth form of the object *a*, we can better see how this relaunching works. Firstly, how does it work in each of the three other forms? Then, how does it work further by itself?

Regarding the first form of the object *a*—the oral object—it is easier to think that we first had something, a concrete reality, of which we are later deprived. It is the same with the real, imaginary and symbolic dimensions. We think we know what they are: a reality. Afterwards comes lack. First paradise, then sin and paradise lost. But we must focus on the very fact that paradise never existed. First sin, first lack, first the radical nothing.

Regarding the second form of the object *a*—the anal object—it is easier to think that the lack, the sin, depends upon us. We could do nothing whilst opposing two concrete forces against each other. But this act—the process of original repression—depends on its triggering by a radical nothing.

In the case of the third form of the object *a*—the scopic object—it is more understandable to think that we already have a ready-made topology, into which we could insert the realistic entities of psychopathology. But psychoanalytic topology is in itself never ready-made. It always supposes the process of questioning the space of encountering the analysand and of the silence entailed in it.

In order to take stock of the issue of the object *a*, we must understand not only the nihilistic character of the radical nothing, but also, more importantly, how it works by itself, even if this work is always reflected in other forms of the object *a*. The question, "How does it work?" is easily understood as, "What are its results?" And then we return again to the first three forms of the object *a*—how the nothing induces us to find a substitute, and this is the treatment of the nothing as oral object. How the nothing can be built as a dialectical opposition between two forces, and that is the analysis of a compromise as anal object. How the nothing of the mapping of the scopic object can be filled up with concrete implementations, and that is the forecasting of the casual difficulties through a given topology aiming to prevent any radical anguish.

However, these different ways of responding to the *object a* are always seen as the result of one of the first three manners of thinking nothing, and conceal the very questioning of the manner itself, of the "how": "How does the nothing work?"

In the French language, we have the equivocation between the noun *faille* which means "failure" and the verb conjugated in the subjunctive present *qu'il faille* which means "it has to be" or "it has to be done." In this equivocation between *faille* and *qu'il faille*, we have a single word for the radical nothing and the core of the practice, without having to explain this through the hazard of practice. This is the momentum of a mere creation, without any regard for the contingency of the world and its demands. The sinthome—that is the best manner to deal with any symptom—consists in this equivocation: sin, failure, the radical nothing and the core of our practice, invention of the sinthome. We must focus on the pure vacuity of the symptom in order to introduce the genuine practice of psychoanalysis, and its acts.

This is precisely the manner of the working of the unconscious. Freud stated at the end of chapter VI of *The Interpretation of Dreams*: "It does not think, calculate or judge in any way at all."[6] In other words, it does not calculate to reach a substi-

6 Freud, S. (1900a). The interpretation of dreams. SE XVII: 507.

tute, it does not think through the analysis of compromises, and does not judge the situation within its mapping in order to prevent difficulties.

"What is it doing then?" A better question is, "How does the unconscious work?" Answer: it invents a new form. The unconscious is essentially ethical, and furthermore, it is the essence of ethics. It is creation. Of course, it uses the material and the matters already present. But it does not care at all about their meaning. It takes any element of these matters—let us write S1—and transforms it as it pleases—let us write S2. This is the essence of the signifier: S1, which is chosen as a stable support (imaginary), S2 and the process of transformation (symbolic), and their mutual articulation (the real). Taking the radical nothing into account leads directly to the signifier and the articulation of imaginary, symbolic and the real in the Borromean chain.

What does this mean for our practice? With evenly suspended attention, we must simultaneously consider: firstly, the imaginary of the chosen matters (what the analysand is speaking about), secondly, the symbolic of the transformation (how it is always moving and changing), and thirdly, the real of what escapes in this entanglement between the imaginary and the symbolic. However, we have neither this Borromean chain nor this evenly suspended attention. We have to create them. We can do this only by taking the radical nothing as the starting point of our invention. We do not have to take into account the theories of Freud or Lacan. But what we do have to take into account is the radical lack. Thus, we have to deal with the appearance of the imaginary, the symbolic, and the real in our listening.

It seems at first that each of these dimensions could exist in itself. But this is not true. For instance, the imaginary of the matters at stake—the symptom—does not exist outside of its formation, as we have seen with psychical reality as explained by Freud. The construction has already started in the symptom, but this implies the engagement of the analyst in his very listening to construct the fourth dimension that holds the three others in a Borromean chain.

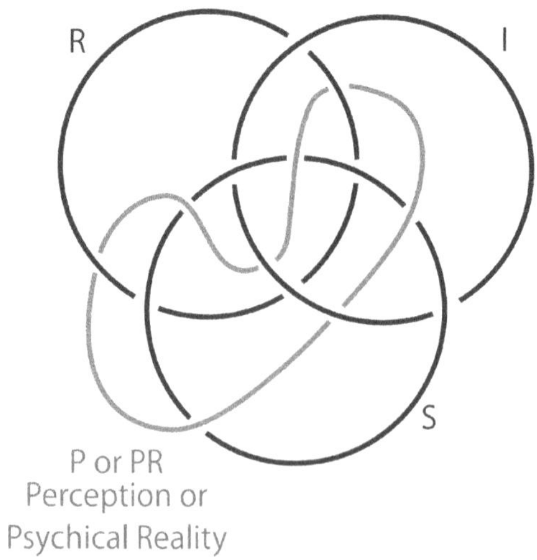

But there is more. Whilst attempting to hold together these three dimensions in a chain, we are necessarily thinking of the continuity of these dimensions, which are transformed into a single rope. This occurs each time we present a clinical case, whilst bringing the imaginary, the symbolic and the real into contact with each other. The case is taken as a unique personality, which is in fact, a paranoid structure, that is, a clover knot.[7]

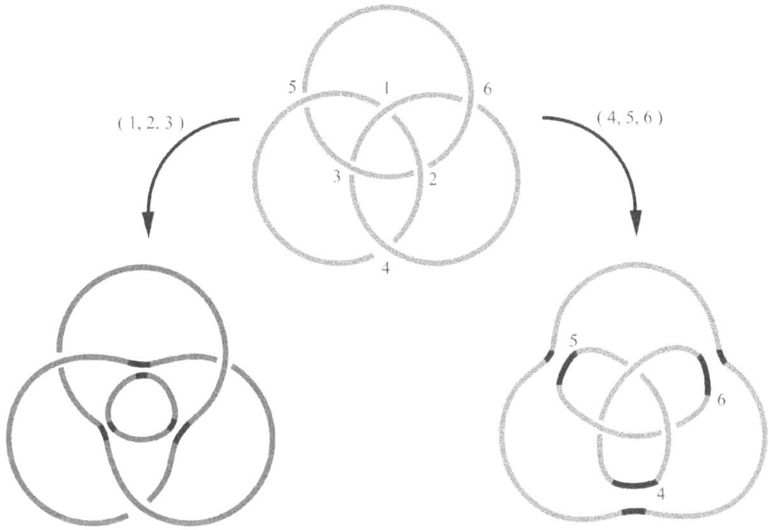

Although we have just one dimension, the entanglement must be kept (as in the figure on the right) and can be lost (as in the figure on the left, which is a trivial round). What does this mean? We must maintain the entanglement, even if we lose the differences between imaginary, symbolic and the real in our presentation of the case as a personality. In order to keep this entanglement, in order to keep track of our evenly suspended attention between these three dimensions, we must repair any failure in the clover knot as soon as it occurs, directly in the place where it occurs.

If our attention is not engaged but merely suspended, we simply let things happen. Of course, sooner or later, we will encounter the entanglement in the phantasm, we will see the psychical reality, and so on. But here we miss the point of the sinthome, its radical failure, and its repair as a creation.

There are two quite different types of psychoanalysis. On the one hand, psychoanalysis can be centred on the phantasm (where we have a mapping of psychic

7 Fierens, C. (2018). *Lecture du sinthome*, p. 128.

reality), and on the other hand, it can be centred on the sinthome, and there, we construct, we invent on the spot with the dynamic unconscious. Such construction is to be started again and again, taking stock of the focus on the radical nothing again and again.

Here we are confronted with an infinite number of traps. For instance, to construct the articulation of the three dimensions, we are accustomed to first articulate two of them, for example, the symbolic and the real. The symbolic is supposed to deal with the real (and we have forgotten the imaginary). So, we form a chain of two components, the symbolic and the real (and the imaginary is lost).

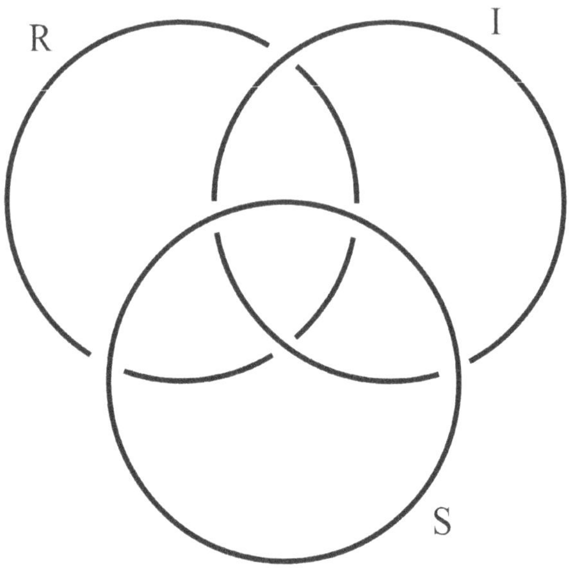

The aim of evenly suspended attention is to keep the imaginary within reach, and, starting from this failure and from the radical nothing, to invent a new form. This is the work of the unconscious. So we must invent a fourth rope, a so-called Ego to keep the imaginary within reach.[8] Then we have to rethink the Ego, narcissism and everything:

8 Fierens, C. (2018). *Lecture du sinthome*, pp. 424–432.

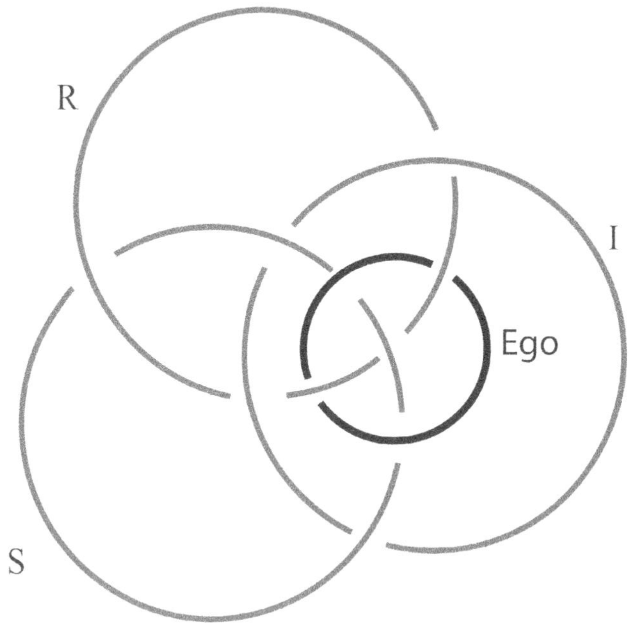

True psychoanalytic topology is not a given in theory. There is no topology in the psychoanalytic field, except that which must be invented in the practice of evenly suspended attention by each analyst. This begins with the object *a*. The fourth form of the object *a*, however, invites us to invent a new form again and again. In this way, it follows the pathway of the unconscious and its symptom or sinthome.

Chapter 28

Enjoyment and sexual disorientation

Christian Fierens

All patients—whether users of health care services or people who frequent social organisations—are aiming to increase their enjoyment, any kind of enjoyment. Nevertheless, enjoyment in general seems doomed to inflict great damage: to the person enjoying (too much enjoyment is bad for the health) as well as to other people (too much enjoyment is bad for justice and the freedom of others), and also to the world at large (too much enjoyment is bad for a sustainable world).

Nowadays, symptoms are confronted more and more with these two sides, this restriction of enjoyment as being much too good or much too bad. Symptoms seek a compromise. The political solution to the question of enjoyment seems to follow this structure of compromise: 'Enjoy yourself, yes. But not too much.' Politics consists in managing enjoyment, that is, in compromising. And this is the first conception of the Freudian symptom.

Confronted with the question of enjoyment, the psychologist, the social worker, the psychiatrist, the psychoanalyst, and so on, seem to have no other alternative than the political one. In other words, they must follow the symptomatic structure, and limit enjoyment or cut it off. As far as jouissance leads to noxious consequences, it must be depreciated, lessened. The positive assessment by the person enjoying must be countered by a negative one, a moderating one. Castration would be the word for such an operation. In this sense, the psychoanalytic worker would follow the general sense of politics and compromise—that is, manage jouissance—for the greatest good of each and every one of us. But such politics does not take into account the very essence of enjoyment.

What is jouissance at its core? Jouissance is often used in the process of a technical action. If we have a goal and we find the means to reach it, we can enjoy the result. In other words, enjoyment would be the subjective result of a technical success. Such technical success can be achieved in any type of action, for instance, a bicycle repair, a good meal, the solution to a mathematics problem, a medical recovery, or even a good action and its reward in heaven. The structure is always the same. In the beginning, we have a situation and a goal in mind, then we use a good technique until we have reached the end point. The schema is: dot arrow dot.

DOI: 10.4324/9781003712480-35

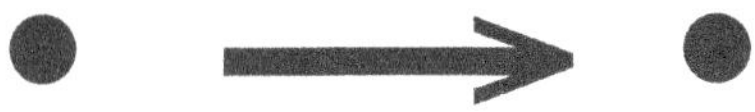

But this technical approach is not sufficient. We must take the subject of the action into account. He—and perhaps somebody else—is pleased with this technical success. Thus, enjoyment is pleasure. Moreover, the pleasure principle generally leads to the reality principle in order to obtain the most sustainable pleasure, whilst taking reality into account. The reality principle is nothing but the continuation of the pleasure principle in reality.

Jouissance is frequently perceived as an immoderate and uncontrolled pleasure; in other words, it does not take reality into account. At the end of the day, such uncontrolled pleasure leads to displeasure, which is the opposite of pleasure. Furthermore, we encounter forms of enjoyment that, rather than seeking pleasure, are directly seeking suffering, pain, death and destruction. We can therefore guess that enjoyment or jouissance is explained neither by a technical principle, nor by the pleasure principle, but by a third principle beyond the pleasure principle, let us say the jouissance principle.

Psychic life: How does it work?		
Technical principle	Pleasure principle (and Reality principle)	Jouissance principle

Three quite different principles—technical, pleasure, and jouissance—determine 'how it works.' These principles do not address the question: what are the results of psychic movement in general, but rather, focus on the very functioning of the symptoms, as well as of every treatment of them and of so-called normal psychic life.

What is to be done? This is precisely Kant's question, on beginning to examine the fundaments of ethics in his *Critique of Practical Reason*. What is to be done? and What are the principles, or what is the principle of ethical action? Following Kant, every human being knows the fact of moral law. This moral law orders without condition. It is a categorical imperative, not a hypothetical one. This means that moral duties are neither determined by any technical purpose, nor for factual pleasure of somebody at a particular moment. These are not hypothetical imperatives. They are not determined by any hypothesis, the hypothesis of a goal to be reached or the hypothesis of happiness to be sought. So, besides the technical principle and the pleasure principle, a third principle must exist—the morality principle—that is categorical and not hypothetical.

What is to be done?		
Hypothetical imperative		Categorical imperative
Technical principle	Pleasure principle (and Reality principle)	Morality principle

In short, let us say that in order to follow this morality principle—in order to be categorical—the moral law must be a formal one, a priori and independent of its enforcement in these matters. To this end, the moral law must conform to three conditions. Firstly, it must be universal: act as if the maxim of your action were to become, through your will, a universal law of nature. Secondly, this law must respect all human beings: act in such a way that you treat humanity—whether in your own person or in the person of any other—never simply as a means, but always, at the same time, as an end. Thirdly, the moral law is not a given, but must be produced. The subject of morality must himself produce the moral law, independently of objects. This autonomy of the moral rule means the possibility of producing it, that is, freedom.

The three formulations of the categorical imperative		
Universality of the law	Respect of human beings	Autonomy and freedom

This type of Kantian morality seems to be completely outdated. It is impossible to find such a moral action corresponding to a true universality, absolutely respecting humanity without any regard for economic factors. It is impossible to find true freedom and a genuine autonomy able to found a true moral law. Moreover, it seems that the Kantian moral law does not exist at all. Indeed, Kant himself wrote that there has probably never been a single completely moral act in the world.

Kantian morality has now faded, and seems to remain an old morality which aims to find happiness through technique. Morality and happiness continue side by side. On the one side, handle things technically as much as you are able, and you will be happy, that is, happiness through morality (the Stoic philosophers). On the other side, take as much pleasure as possible in everything, enjoy yourself, have fun, and you will realise yourself, that is, morality through happiness (the Epicurean philosophers).

Stoic morality	Epicurean morality
Means: morality	Means: pleasure
Goal: happiness	Goal: morality

With these two moralities, the technical principle and the pleasure principle are entangled. Even if the presence of other people is taken into account, there remains no place for a third principle. In politics, other people are still managed with the technical principle and the pleasure principle.

Nevertheless, in daily life and in our practice we endlessly encounter guilt, culpability. If we think only in terms of the first two principles, it is easy to manage this culpability and to say such things as: 'This is the failure of the two aforementioned principles,' 'You are guilty because you did it wrongly, because you handled the technique badly,' or 'You are guilty because you missed the point, because you didn't attain happiness.' This is the usual way of treating psychological disorders. The technical education of the child was not good. The parents did it wrongly. They are to be blamed. They are guilty. At the same time, the patient must also be blamed, because he does not want to attain pleasure. The patient's defence—his negative therapeutic reaction—is due to his bad will.

With such modes of thinking—arguments restraining psychic life to technique and to the seeking of happiness—what is striking is that the treatment remains completely ineffective. Moreover, the culpability of the parents and of the patient is then doubled down with the culpability of the psychotherapist, who has failed to cure the patient and is unhappy about this. We have reached the complete standoff of both principles: technical and pleasure. What remains is guilt.

But what is the essence of guilt or of culpability? Guilt is impossible to delete. It remains year after year after the crime, even if one attempts to repair the original failure, even if time has tried to buffer the gravity of the failure, even if the fault is forgiven and forgotten. Even if the fault was a tiny one or even an imaginary one, culpability remains. Moreover, culpability was probably already present before the crime was committed. For example, a potential criminal might be assailed by unconscious feelings of guilt—before seeking a reason for this culpability and before finding this reason—whilst committing a crime. So, there would be guilt long before and long after the crime, above and beyond—as well as beneath—the functioning of the technical and pleasure principles.

What is guilt? Guilt is precisely the reverse side of the moral act. We never found the Kantian moral act. But we are always found guilty. We do not find the recto of moral acts, only the verso in the culpability.

What is to be done?		
Hypothetical imperative		Categorical imperative
Technical principle	Pleasure principle (and Reality principle)	(Morality principle) Guilt Culpability

Let us try to catch a glimpse of this fundamental verso side, of the essential guilt, the original sin. To explain his method at the beginning of *The Interpretation of Dreams*, Freud relates his own dream of Irma's injection.[1] Freud had made medical mistakes with his patient Irma. He is guilty. The meaning of the dream is a wish fulfilment and this fulfilment sounds like: 'he (Freud) is not guilty.' Could all dreams be about culpability?

Not Guilty	Guilty
Wish fulfilment	Culpability
Pleasure principle	Beyond the pleasure principle: The jouissance principle

Let us leave this question for a moment and refer to the end of Chapter VI, where Freud emphasises that the functioning of the unconscious in the dream "does not think, calculate or judge in any way at all."[2] Here is my comment about this statement of Freud's: the unconscious does not care about thinking about pleasure, about calculating the technical process to reach the goal, about judging practically what is to be done in order to obey a technical principle, or a pleasure principle. The working of the unconscious merely restricts itself to transforming.

What does this mean, this restriction to transforming, to giving things a new form? Could this new form have any form whatsoever, a random one? If this were so, the working of the unconscious would lead step by step to complete mayhem. But this is not the case. So how is it possible to give a new form independently of the matter, that is, independently of the things to be thought about, to be calculated with, and to be judged upon?

Giving a form independently of the matter is precisely the Kantian questioning on morality. The unconscious gives a new form quite independently of the matter and its hypothesis, and this is the same with the Kantian moral law. The unconscious transformation must be done without condition: it works as a categorical imperative. The status of the unconscious is an ethical one, corresponding more precisely to the Kantian one. Furthermore, as the moral act that is never fulfilled, the unconscious never reaches the fulfilment of its categorical imperative. Thus, it produces guilt and culpability far more than it produces wish fulfilment. The fulfilment in Freud's dream of Irma's injection seems to be the acquittal of his fault ('he is not guilty'), but in doing so, simultaneously emphasises the unforgivable fault—the original sin—that is the starting point of his dream. And here I add: this original sin can now become the starting point of another invention.

From the beginning, we must consider psychoanalysis in regard to the unconscious, which responds neither to a technical principle, nor to the pleasure principle. As demands remain stuck in technical problems and pleasure seeking, we must

1 Freud, S. (1900a). The method of interpreting dreams: An analysis of a specimen dream. In: *The Interpretation of Dreams*. SE IV: 107.

2 Freud, S. (1900a). The dream-work. In: *The Interpretation of Dreams*. SE IV: 507.

keep the logic of the demand at bay. We must deal with a third principle beyond the pleasure principle—the jouissance principle—which responds to a structure similar to the Kantian categorical imperative. This would reach the universality of a natural law, it would like to completely respect human beings, and has to be done in the autonomy of the unconscious. But each time it fails, it remains contingent, scorns human essence and delays its action. So, the dynamic unconscious does not produce an accomplished moral act as Kantian morality intended to do, but rather, its failure, that is, culpability. Let us try not to alleviate the weight of culpability as in the case of Freud in his dream of Irma's injection. Rather, let us take stock of this a priori fault to keep in touch with the unconscious work, its ethical status and its failure. Then we can invent and create with the unconscious.

This is easy to say. But regularly, and necessarily, the old logic of the first two principles regains the upper hand. In regard to the unconscious, we are prone to thinking that we have a given person, a so-called subject who has to choose between different possible actions, with a goal to be reached. What is the best action here? Where is the Good? Only afterwards, and secondarily, would we need to take stock of the difficulties arising from the unconscious. There is a similar misunderstanding regarding Kantian morality: we are prone to consider it a treaty for given human subjects who must choose between different possible actions. Which is the best one? Where is the Good? The answer would be the criterion of a given universality, the rule of universality.

With regard to the conception of the unconscious as well as that of Kantian morality, the reality of the subject and the reality of the Good are two fundamental mistakes. Firstly, we do not have a given subject. Regarding the unconscious, the subject is only a result, the effect of a process implying the unconscious. We never have a subject who begins a speech on his own. It is the unconscious in each discourse that starts the whole process. Regarding Kantian morality, in the dialectic or his first *Critique*, *Critique of Pure Reason*, Kant emphasised that the subject, the so-called soul, is a mere illusion, a paralogism.[3] It is only within the questioning of his second *Critique*, *Critique of Practical Reason*, that the subject can acquire an existence. In its existence, the subject is completely dependent on ethics, and not the contrary.[4]

Secondly, we do not have the Good, as an aim for a morality that would be the technique to reach the Good. The Good is a pure Platonic idea without any accessible reality, except as the result of a relative success of the technique or the relative pleasure of a fulfilled wish in a dream.

We are necessarily entangled in these two misunderstandings. We always believe in a primary subject, in the person. We always believe in a Good, which would be

3 Kant, I. (1998 [1781]). *The Cambridge Edition of the Works of Immanuel Kant: Critique of Pure Reason*. Cambridge: Cambridge University Press.

4 Kant, I. (1996 [1788]). Critique of practical reason. In: *The Cambridge Edition of the Works of Emmanuel Kant: Practical Philosophy*. Cambridge: Cambridge University Press, pp. 133–271.

worthy of the general aim for our actions. So, if we want to keep in touch with the dynamic of the unconscious—with ethics congruent with the Kantian practical question—we must deal with these two misunderstandings of a given subject and of a given Good.

Lacan obviously misunderstands Kantian morality, or, at least he feigns misunderstanding it. Regardless, in his essay Kant with Sade, Lacan corrects this misunderstanding with the help of Sade. Thus he gives us a pathway to find what he calls 'the Kant truth' and, at the same time, a pathway to keep in touch with the very functioning of the unconscious.

To counter the so-called Kantian morality of a subject aiming at the Good, Lacan introduces Sadean morality, aiming at Evil and the destruction of the subject. Confronting Good and Evil only opens the pathway to the Real, which is far beyond Good and Evil (Nietzsche). To counter the primarily-given subject, Lacan introduces the destruction of the subject in Sadean stages. Such destruction is at stake in the process of any phantasm. Each phantasm is not only an image of subjective activities, but also entails the radical questioning of the subject, more specifically, the destruction of the subject as it was commonly accepted by the subject himself and by society.

These two points have practical consequences for psychoanalytic practice. Firstly, in regard to the position towards Good and Evil: if the analyst does not suggest an ideal of Good and if he does not try to avoid Evil for the analysand, this is not purely abstinence, but is for the active introduction to the Real or to the functioning of the unconscious principle, that is, the jouissance principle. We will see how. Secondly, in regard to the position towards the subject: if the analyst takes stock of the phantasm and its process, it is not in order to reach a better identification of the subject. On the contrary, this is in order to relaunch a questioning while destroying this subjective identification.

But what is the pathway of this questioning of the subject and of the introduction to the Real? Here the three formulae of the Kantian categorical imperative can help. Firstly, act as if the maxim of your action were to become, through your will, a universal law of nature. 'As if,' 'act as if:' the Kant universality is neither a rule, nor a given law, but an 'as if.' The Real is not a given, nor is it made by us. We can approach it only with our 'as if': as if it were beyond every condition. This aims to put aside the pragmatic conditions of the action. If you must choose something very important in your life—for example, a life partner or a profession—do not think about the pragmatic conditions. Do not calculate its price. Do not judge its consequences. If you must deal with the unconscious, do not think about the phenomenal conditions. Do not calculate its price. Do not judge the consequences. Act as if you were creating a new law, a new form in nature. This is the very functioning of the unconscious.

Secondly, act in such a way that you always treat humanity—whether in your own person or in the person of any other—not simply as a means, but always, at the same time, as an end. Treating human beings as human means to take the human into account, not simply as a means, as an imaginary element for any intention, but also, and not least of all, as an end. But the end of the human being is death—the big gap—which focuses the whole symbolic process. It is quite impossible to master, at the same time, the human as a means and the human as an end, as Kant seemed to think. It is impossible to master, at the same time, the imaginary point of view of the means for pragmatic actions and the symbolic point of view of the end of human beings. This impossibility leads precisely towards the Real.

Thirdly, the moral law is not a given, but must be produced. The subject of morality must himself produce the moral law. This autonomy of the moral rule means the possibility of producing it, that is, freedom. We can approach the Real only if we accept to do, that is, if we start from the radical nothing—from the original sin, from the first failure—and if we are confronted with its invitation to create and to invent. This is the sense of the Lacanian sinthome.

To take stock of the unconscious and of the jouissance principle, it is necessary to disclose the failure, the original sin, the radical nothing—the core of guilt—which is concealed behind the multitude of technical activities and the infinite hopes of happiness: I am in the place from which the universe is a flaw in the purity of Non-being is vociferated. And not without reason for, by protecting itself, this place makes being itself languish (l-a-n-g-i-s-h). This place is called jouissance, and it is jouissance whose absence would render the universe vain.[5]

Where is this place of jouissance? It is everywhere. Nowadays, the word of enjoyment—its technical principles and its aim, towards limitless pleasure—overwhelms the world. It seems that there is no place for the purity of Non-being, in other words, for the radical nothing or for the vocal form of Lacan's object *a*.

This usual topic of enjoyment—with its technique, pleasure, pain and destruction—conceals the jouissance principle, the unconscious principle, the purity of non-being. Nevertheless, the non-being does not fail to appear as culpability, as failure, as guilt. Ashamed about this failure, we attempt to avoid it. Taken in the contemporary manner of thinking, we are prone to submit this failure to technique in order to erase the culpability, to forget it and return to the technical actions aiming at happiness. Even in the psychoanalytic field, we frequently find enquiries which aim in this direction: to explain that it is 'not your fault,' that it is 'not so bad,' or that it is only an imaginary fault. But we must take stock of the fact that culpability gives us a first glimpse of the very place of the analyst in his discourse—the place of semblance of the object *a*, of a nothing but a radical nothing—the sin giving access to the invention of the sinthome.

Thus, we must take common enjoyment into account as a first step towards the jouissance principle, all the more so since this common enjoyment, in its insistence, conceals the purity of non-being and in concealing it, reveals its truth.

5 Lacan, J. (1977 [1966]). The subversion of the subject and the dialectic of desire in the Freudian unconscious. In: *Écrits: A Selection*. A. Sheridan (Trans.). New York & London: Norton & Co., pp. 292–325.

Starting from this radical nothing, can we find a so-called orientation that would answer the question once and for all: what is to be done? What is to be done will always be done with interest. And interest is fundamentally sexual. To answer the question, what is to be done? we must take stock of sexuality or libido. And this, we know, is always focused on the phallus. There is only one type of libido, for men and women. For all, the phallus is at stake: "for all x phi of x."[6] Here it seems that we find ourselves back at the first formulation of Kant's moral law—universality as the given phallic function valid for everybody—as well as the second, the real essence of human beings, the phallic essence, to be respected. Thus we have the group of all human beings with this universal phallic function.

But as for any group, there must be a leader—a person or an idea, it doesn't matter—and we think that this leader would be an exception, the founder of the phallic function in the figure of the father, who would be outside the phallic function: "there exists an x not phi of x."[7] This figure is whoever has created the phallic law. Such creation corresponds to the third formulation of Kant's moral law. But watch out! In Kant's law, the creator or the maker of the law is the subject of the law himself. It is the so-called autonomy entailing the freedom of the subject. In the classical explanation of the phallic function, this is not the subject himself but the father. The creator of the law is outside of the subject. He is not subjected to the phallic law.

Given these two formulae, we have an orientation to distinguish two types of human beings: the followers or the subjects who try to obey the phallic law, and the leaders, the ideal figures representing the Good, those who create the law and enforce it upon others.

But beware! If we lose autonomy and freedom, we also lose the structure of Kantian morality, as well as the structure of the unconscious which does not think, does not calculate, does not judge at all. If thinking, calculating and judging accord with the father, who impersonates the big Other, then with this father figure, we also lose the third principle: the morality principle or the jouissance principle. Everything is working following the technique that is aimed at the father. Hopefully, the father would be the guarantor of our happiness, of subjects and of the Good.

But this is not true. There is a fundamental failure—the original sin—that appears with the first woman. The subject does not exist as such but is simply a fiction that depends upon a working process that existed long before its appearance. We think that we have subjects, because they are stuck in our theory—in the phallic function, for instance—dependent on the Good represented by the father. The so-called reality of these subjects must be destroyed by phantasmic questioning, because the big Other does not exist. We must take into account the fact that "there

6 Lacan, J. (2013 [1971–1972]). *The Knowledge of the Psychoanalyst/Le Savoir du Psychanalyste*. M. G. Plastow (Trans.). Saint-Denis: l'Association Lacanienne Internationale (for private use only).

7 Lacan, J. (2013 [1971–1972]). *The Knowledge of the Psychoanalyst.*

does not exist an x not phi of x."[8] The sin is not the sin of the feminine woman, but is the sin of the Good itself—of God—of the big Other.

As a consequence, the phallic function is not founded at all, and the so-called subjects of the law cannot remain stuck in their phallic functioning: "not all phi of x."[9] But this formula is not only a negative one. Orphans of the big Other—who does not exist—have to make on their own, without him. They? Who? The remnants of the so-called subject: unconscious elements. And this is the creation of the unconscious inventing a new form, as well as the creation of the law in its autonomy.

It seems that, starting from the questioning—how does it work? or what is to be done?—with the third principle, we have found the four formulae of the phallic function or the four formulae of sexuation:

Sexuation or phallic function	*Subject*	*Good*
Male	for all x phi of x	there exists an x not phi of x
Female	not all phi of x	there does not exist an x not phi of x

In this summary table, which must be critiqued, we see that the two feminine formulae represent the contradiction of the supposed subject and of the supposed Good exception of the masculine formulae. Destruction of the subject and of the Good was precisely the way to keep in touch with the jouissance principle of the unconscious, as well as with genuine Kantian morality. Lacan used Sade's literary works in this sense.

Now, with this table, we have different manners of answering the question: what is to be done? We have seen the so-called masculine manners, divided between the leaders and the followers. And we can add the so-called feminine manners, which would be divided between the leaders' opponents and the followers' opponents. This would provide us with a beautiful schema for the possible sexual orientations of the subject. We could identify the human subject as masculine or as feminine, and inside each of them, an identification as leader, representing the Good, or as subject of the law.

But such orientations with the formulae of sexuation completely miss the point of the very questioning of the unconscious and its jouissance principle. These orientations suppose that the entries in the table exist as a reality: the reality of the subject and the reality of the Good, the realities of males and females. But this is not the case, as they always depend on the process of the dynamic unconscious.

8 Lacan, J. (2013 [1971–1972]). *The Knowledge of the Psychoanalyst.*
9 Lacan, J. (2013 [1971–1972]). *The Knowledge of the Psychoanalyst.*

Therefore, to explain the formulae, we must take up a different point of view. This process implies not only the four formulae, but importantly, their roundabout in the same process. It is impossible to consider one single formula independently of the others. The schema would be something like this:

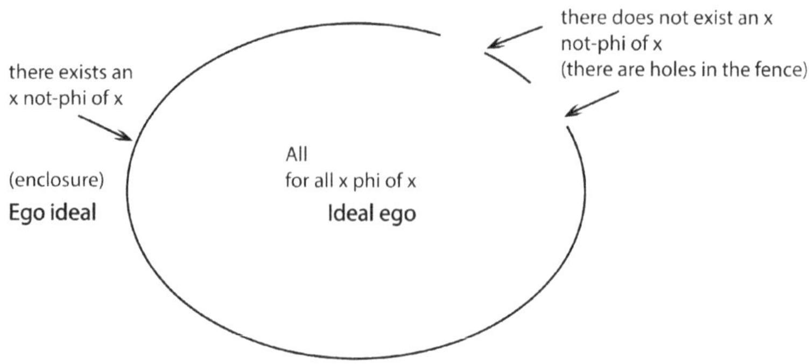

With this schema, we do not have any sexual orientations in which to identify the subject. That would be sexuality. Rather, we would have disorientation—a principle of continually questioning sexuality—which means making sexuality anew, in other words, a sexuation. This is not a matter of obeying a given orientation, but of questioning any orientation. It is such disorientation that keeps the sexuation alive.

Of course, any enjoyment can be understood as a given symptomatology. Even if the process is concealed, however, it permits a glimpse of the place of Non-being—of the radical nothing—of the opening up to creation, beginning from the unconscious. The place of the analyst is one that takes this Non-being—this radical nothing—into account. It is the place of the analyst, therefore, that opens the field to the jouissance principle. Moreover, this does not follow the subject, or the Good, but starts from their failure. Let us hope that we can hear the disorientation of the unconscious and a new sexuation at the core of any jouissance.

Index

For Product Safety Concerns and Information please contact our EU representative GPSR@taylorandfrancis.com
Taylor & Francis Verlag GmbH, Kaufingerstraße 24, 80331 München, Germany

www.ingramcontent.com/pod-product-compliance
Ingram Content Group UK Ltd.
Pitfield, Milton Keynes, MK11 3LW, UK
UKHW021724240926
475702UK00030BA/2548
9781041196068